WORKED PROBLEMS IN VIS[...]

Errors and omissions

Q14 $$y = p\left|\dfrac{K}{K'}\right|$$ $$y = 4\left|\dfrac{-6}{54}\right| = 0.\dot{4}mm$$ $$\therefore \left|h'_u\right| + y = 1.295 + 0.\dot{4} = 1.739mm$$	**Q16[b][i]** $$y = p\left|\dfrac{K}{K'}\right|$$ $$y = 4\left|\dfrac{4.69}{55.31}\right| = 0.339mm$$
Q17[ii] $$y = p\left|\dfrac{K}{K'}\right|$$ $$y = 3\left|\dfrac{7}{67}\right| = 0.313mm$$	**Q20** $$k' = 3.6 + 3.6 + 16.97 = 24.17$$ $$\therefore K' = +55.16$$ $$\therefore h'_u = -\dfrac{1}{K'}\tan\omega°$$ $$\therefore h'_u = -\dfrac{1}{55.16}\tan 5° = -1.57mm$$
Q21[ii] Should read $-5.00DS$ lens @ 12mm	**Q23[c]** h'_u as well as h'_c should be negative
Q22[b] h'_u should be negative as should h'_c in [c] & [d]	**Q43[b]** Find the retinal image size for an object 5mm high situated at near point.
Q31[b] $$F_{sp} = -3.00D$$ $$f'_{sp} = 100/-3$$ $$= -33.33cm$$ $$d = 1.5cm$$ $$\therefore k = -34.83cm$$ $$\therefore K = 100/-34.83$$ $$= -2.87D$$ $$F_e = +60.00D$$ $$\overline{K'} = -2.87 + 60 = +57.13D$$ $$k' = 4/3 \times 1000/57.13$$ $$= +23.34mm$$ In the aphakic eye $$k' = 23.34 + 1.68 = 25.02mm$$ $$\overline{K'} = 4/3 \times 1000/25.02 = +53.29D$$ $$r_c = 7.55mm$$ $$\therefore F_e = \dfrac{1000 \times (\frac{4}{3}-1)}{7.55} = +44.15D$$	**Q31 continued** $$\therefore K - F_e = +53.29 - 44.15 = +9.14D$$ $$\therefore k = \dfrac{1000}{K} = 109.41mm$$ New $d = 15 - 1.68 = 13.32mm$ $$F = \dfrac{K}{1+dK}$$ $$\therefore F = \dfrac{9.14}{1+0.01332 \times 9.14} = +8.15DS$$ power of spectacle lens $= +8.15DS$
	Q53b) $$y = p\left|\dfrac{K'-L'}{K'}\right| = 2\left|\dfrac{57-59.83}{57}\right| = +0.099mm$$ (d) Should read – If this eye is corrected by a lens at 15mm, calculate......
	Q65 should read – A 1cm high object is placed 35cm from the lens.....
	Q73 A printing error has displaced – from 8.00D

WORKED PROBLEMS IN VISUAL OPTICS

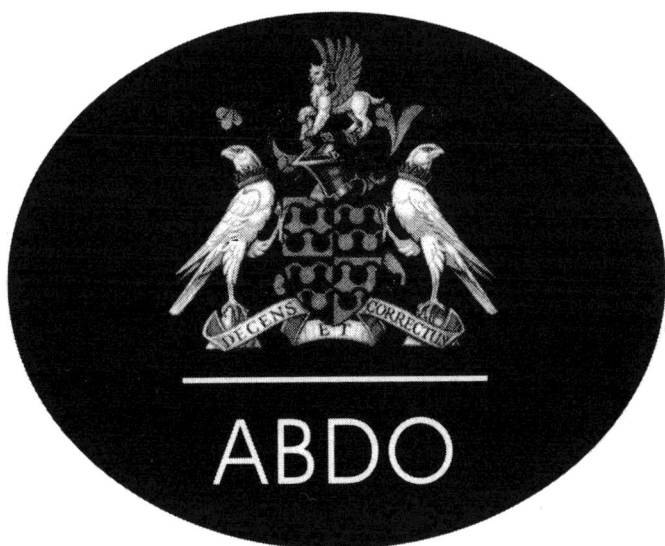

ABDO

By

Tony Griffiths

Published by:

ABDO College of Education
Godmersham Park
Godmersham
Canterbury
Kent
CT4 7DT

ISBN 0-900099-31-3

First Edition   1998
Reprinted   2003

Printed by 4edge Limited

My grateful thanks go to Gordon Hirst for his untiring work in proof reading and correcting my efforts on this and many other occasions.

It almost amounted to major surgery this time!

INDEX

*More than one topic may appear in any worked problem

1. The length of an axially hypermetropic eye is 19*mm*. Find the power of the thin correcting lens placed at 10*mm* from the principal point of the reduced eye.

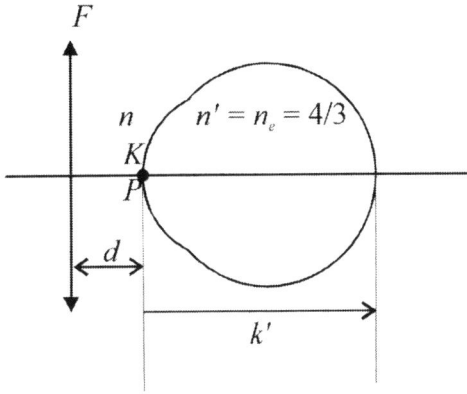

Axial length of eye
$$k' = +0.019m$$

Power of the eye
$$F_e = +60D$$

Vertex distance
$$d = 0.010m$$

Refractive index of eye
$$n_e = 4/3$$

$$\overline{K}' = \frac{n_e}{k'} = \frac{4/3}{+0.019} = +70.18D$$

$$K = \overline{K}' - F_e = (+70.18) - (+60) = +10.18D$$

$$F = \frac{K}{1+dK} = \frac{10.18}{1+0.010\times10.18} = +9.24D$$

2. The far point of a hypermetropic reduced eye is 17*cm* from the principal point. What is the power of the correcting lens at 12*mm*?

$k = +0.17m \quad d = 0.012m$

$K = \dfrac{1}{k} = \dfrac{1}{0.17} = +5.88D$

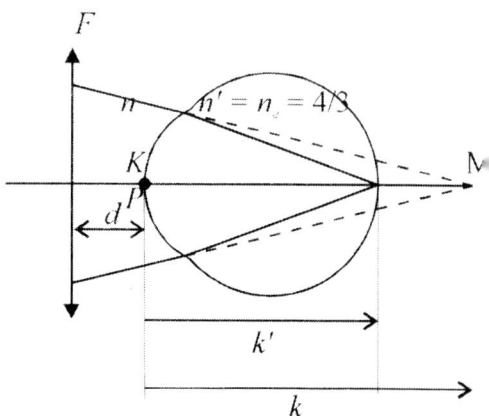

$F = \dfrac{K}{1+dK} = \dfrac{5.88}{1+0.012 \times 5.88} = +5.49D$

> **3.** A myopic eye is corrected with a thin –6.00D lens at 12*mm*. Find the position of the far point. What would be the power of the lens if it were to be dispensed at 15*mm*?

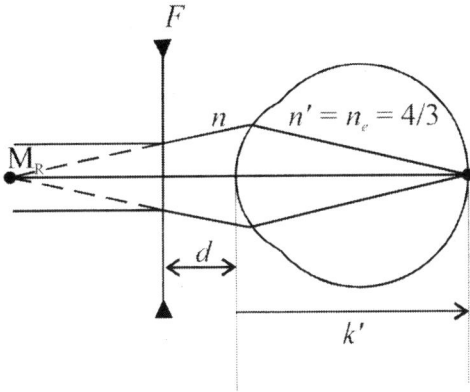

Power of lens at cornea K

$$K = \frac{F}{1 - dF}$$

$$K = \frac{-6}{1 - 0.012 \times (-6)}$$

$$K = \frac{-6}{1.072} = -5.60D$$

Far point $= \dfrac{1}{K} = -178.571mm$

$$F_n = \frac{F_o}{1 + (d_n - d_o)F_o}$$

$$F_n = \frac{-6}{1 + (0.015 - 0.012)(-6)}$$

$$F_n = -6.11D$$

4. The ocular refraction of a myopic eye is numerically 8.00D. Find the power of the correcting spectacle lens worn at 15mm from the reduced surface.

$K = -8.00D$

$d = 0.015m$

$$F_v' = \frac{K}{1 + dK}$$

$$F_v' = \frac{-8}{1 + 0.015 \times -8}$$

$$F_v' = -9.09D$$

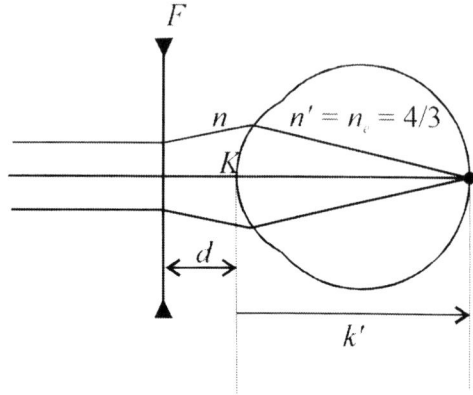

5. An axial object point is half a metre from an axially myopic eye. If a $-3D$ lens is placed in contact with the eye a clear retinal image is formed in the unaccommodated eye. Find the ocular refraction and the axial length of the reduced eye.

$$L = \frac{1}{\ell} = \frac{1}{-0.5} = -2D$$

$$L' = F + L$$
$$= -3 + (-2) = -5D$$

$$K = L' = -5D$$

$$\overline{K}' = K + F_e = -5 + 60 = +55$$

$$k' = \frac{n_e}{\overline{K}'} = \frac{4/3}{+55} = +0.024242m$$
$$= 24.242mm$$

6. [a] Describe the relationship between ocular refraction and spectacle refraction with the help of the expression $f' = k + d$, and a diagram.

[b] Explain the effects when a $-12.00DS$ correction prescribed to be worn at a vertex distance of $10mm$ is dispensed at a vertex distance of $15mm$.

[a]

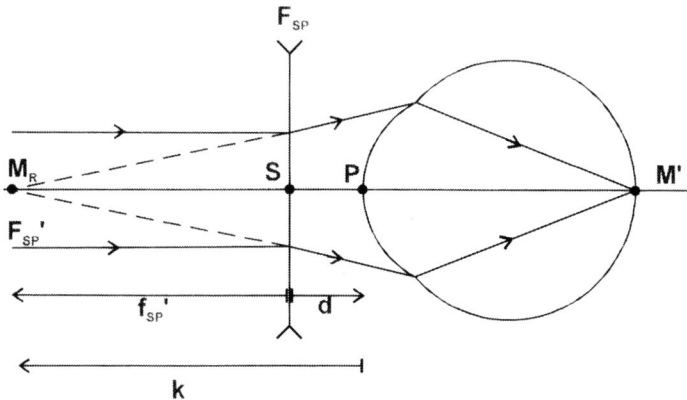

From the diagram, the following equation can be deduced: [remembering sign convention].

$$-k = -f' + d$$
$$\therefore f' = k + d \qquad \qquad \qquad \qquad \qquad \qquad ①$$

Taking reciprocals for both sides gives:

$$\frac{1}{f'} = \frac{1}{(k+d)}$$

For a thin lens in air, $F = \dfrac{1}{f'}$ [where F = spectacle refraction]

Also: $K = \dfrac{1}{k}$ [where K = ocular refraction]

Hence: $F = \dfrac{1}{(k+d)}$

Substituting $K = \dfrac{1}{k}$ gives: $F = \dfrac{K}{(1+dK)}$

Re-arranging for K gives $K = \dfrac{F}{(1-dF)}$

This equation bears direct comparison with the effective power equation

$$F_x = \dfrac{F}{(1-dF)}$$

where F_x represents the effective power, or effectivity of a thin lens at a distance d to the right of the lens.

Hence, the ocular refraction is the effective power of the spectacle lens at the reduced surface, to render the eye emmetropic.

[b] Using the equation from [a] $K = \dfrac{F}{(1-dF)}$:

When the $-12.00DS$ is worn @ 10mm,

$$K = \dfrac{-12}{(1-\{0.01 \times -12\})} = -10.71D$$

When the $-12.00DS$ is worn @ 15mm,

$$K = \frac{-12}{\left(1 - \{0.015 \times -12\}\right)}$$

$$K = \frac{-12}{1.18} = -10.17D$$

From these two values for K, it can be seen that, if the correction is worn $5mm$ further from the eye than prescribed, there is an effective decrease in power in the case of a minus lens which would be noticed by the patient.

7. A reduced eye with axial hypermetropia is corrected with a thin +6.00DS lens at 15mm. Calculate the ocular refraction and axial length of the eye.

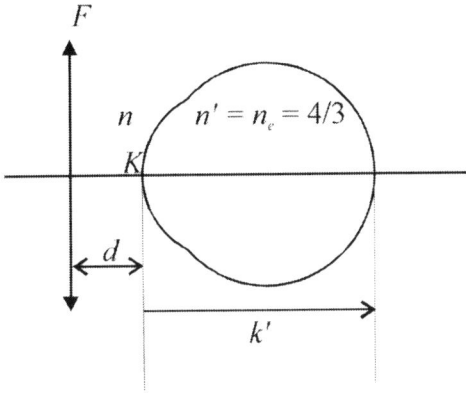

Using $K = \dfrac{F}{(1-dF)}$

$$K = \frac{+6}{(1-0.015\times6)} = \frac{+6}{(1-0.09)}$$

$$\therefore K = +6.59D$$

To find the axial length, first find $\overline{K}'$ from $K = \overline{K}' - F_e$

Where $F_e = +60DS$ since the eye is axially ametropic.

$$\therefore \overline{K}' = K + F_e = +6.59 + 60 = +66.59D$$

$$k' = \frac{n'}{K'}$$

$$\therefore k' = \frac{4/3}{+66.59} = 0.020023m$$

$\therefore$ Axial length of the eye is 20.023mm

8. A lens with parameters $F_1 = +10.50D$, $F_2 = -6.00D$, $t = 7mm$ and refractive index 1.523 corrects an eye for distance vision when fitted at 11mm. Calculate the ocular refraction.

$F_1 = +10.50D$ $F_2 = -6.00D$

$t = 0.007m$

$\bar{t} = 0.004596m$

$d = 0.011m$

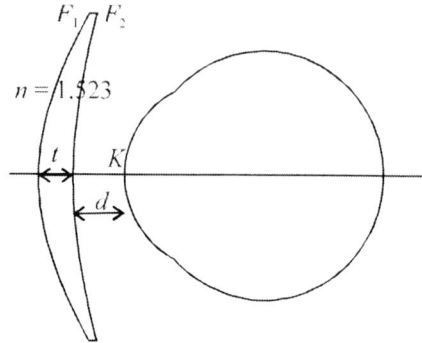

$$F_v' = \frac{F_1 + F_2 - \bar{t}F_1F_2}{1 - \bar{t}F_1}$$

$$F_v' = \frac{+10.5 - 6 - 0.004596 \times 10.5 \times -6}{1 - 0.004596 \times 10.5}$$

$$F_v' = +5.03D$$

$$K = \frac{F_v'}{1 - dF_v'} = \frac{+5.03}{1 - 0.011 \times 5.03} = +5.33D$$

9. An uncorrected myopic reduced eye of axial length 25*mm* views a distant object subtending 5°. If n_e = 1.3333, find the retinal image size.

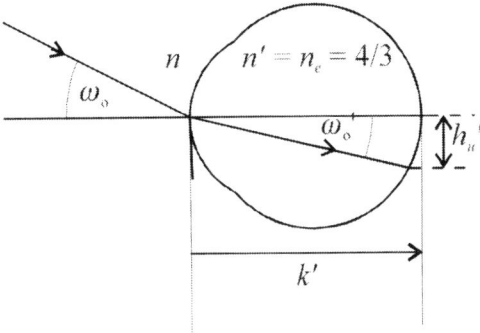

Since h_u' is proportional to k', the longer the axial length the larger will be the uncorrected image size.

$$h_u' = -\frac{k'}{n_e}\tan\omega_o$$

$$h_u' = -\frac{1}{1.3333}k'\tan w_o$$

$$h_u' = -\frac{1}{1.3333}\times 0.025\tan 5$$

$$h_u' = -0.001640m$$

10. In question 9, find the ocular refraction and the thin spectacle lens power if the latter is worn at 14*mm*.

$$k' = +0.025m$$

$$\overline{K}' = \frac{n_e}{k'} = \frac{1.3333}{0.025} = +53.33D$$

$$K = \overline{K}' - F_e = (+53.33) - (+60) = -6.67D$$

$$F = \frac{K}{1+dK} = \frac{-6.67}{1+0.014\times -6.67} = -7.36D$$

11. The far point of a hypermetropic reduced eye is 19cm from the principal point. What is the power of the correcting lens at 15mm?

$$K = \frac{1}{k} = \frac{1}{+0.19} = +5.26D$$

$$F = \frac{K}{1 + dK}$$

$$F = \frac{5.26}{1 + 0.015 \times 5.26}$$

$$F = +4.88D$$

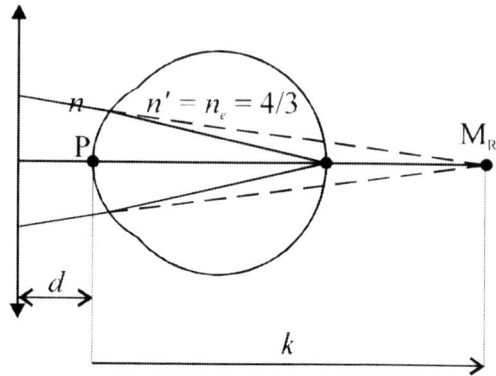

---

12. A thick lens with $F_1 = +10.50D$, $F_2 = -4D$, $t = 9mm$ and $n = 1.71$ is fitted at $9mm$. Find the power of the front surface of the lens if the lens is fitted at $16mm$, the other parameters remaining the same.

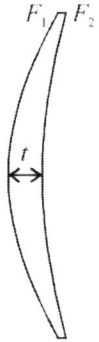

First we must find the Back Vertex Power from

$$\bar{t} = \frac{9}{1.71} = 5.263mm$$

$$F_v' = \frac{F_1 + F_2 - \bar{t}F_1F_2}{1 - \bar{t}F_1}$$

$$F_v' = \frac{+10.5 + (-4) - 0.005263 \times 10.5 \times (-4)}{1 - 0.005263 \times 10.5}$$

$$F_v' = \frac{6.72}{0.945} = +7.11D$$

Next we need to find the Back Vertex Power required at the new distance of $16mm$ from:

$$F_n = \frac{F_o}{1 + (d_n - d_o)F_o}$$

$$F_n = \frac{7.11}{1 + (0.016 - 0.009)7.11}$$

$$F_n = +6.77D$$

Finally we can calculate the compensated front surface power from:

$$F_1 = \frac{F_v' - F_2}{1 + \bar{t}(F_v' - F_2)}$$

$$F_1 = \frac{6.77 - (-4)}{1 + 0.005263(10.77)}$$

$$F_1 = +10.19D$$

13

13. Calculate the blur circle diameters for a distant axial object point when the ocular refraction of 5D is due to [a] axial myopia, [b] refractive myopia, [c] axial hypermetropia and [d] refractive hypermetropia. Assume a pupil diameter of 4mm at the reduced surface.

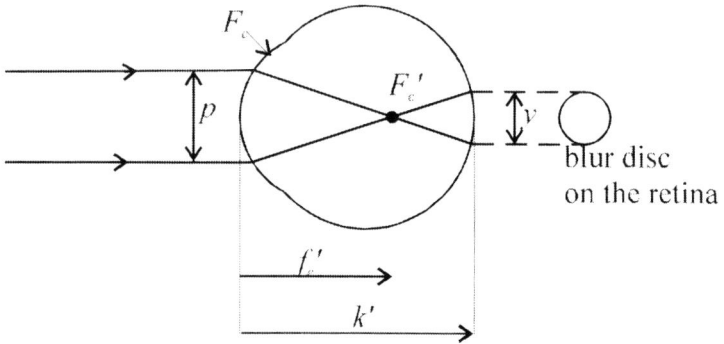

blur disc
on the retina

[a]

$$\overline{K}' = K + F_e$$
$$\overline{K}' = (-5) + 60 = +55D$$

$$y = p\left[\frac{K}{\overline{K}'}\right]$$

$$y = 4\left[\frac{-5}{55}\right] = -0.\dot{3}\dot{6}mm$$

[b] With refractive myopia $\overline{K}' = +60D$

$$y = p\left[\frac{K}{\overline{K}'}\right]$$

$$y = 4\left[\frac{-5}{60}\right] = -0.\dot{3}mm$$

14

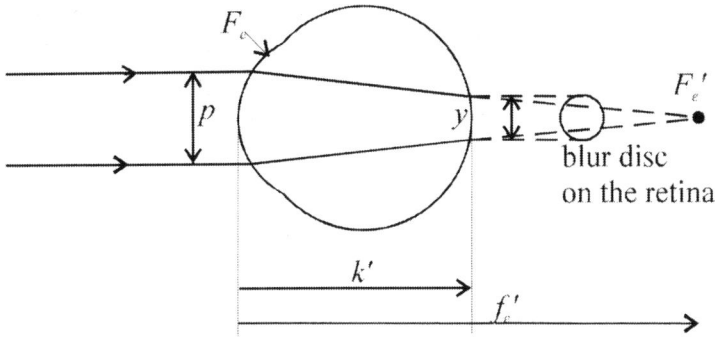

blur disc
on the retina

[c]

$$\overline{K}' = K + F_e$$

$$\overline{K}' = +5 + 60 = +65D$$

$$y = p\left[\frac{K}{\overline{K}'}\right]$$

$$y = 4\left[\frac{+5}{65}\right] = +0.308mm$$

[d] As with refractive myopia $\overline{K}' = +60D$

$$y = p\left[\frac{K}{\overline{K}'}\right]$$

$$y = 4\left[\frac{+5}{60}\right] = +0.\dot{3}mm$$

14. An uncorrected axially myopic eye with $K = -6D$ views a distant object subtending $4°$. If the pupil diameter is $4mm$, find the retinal image size in the uncorrected eye (h_u') and the total extent of the blurred image.

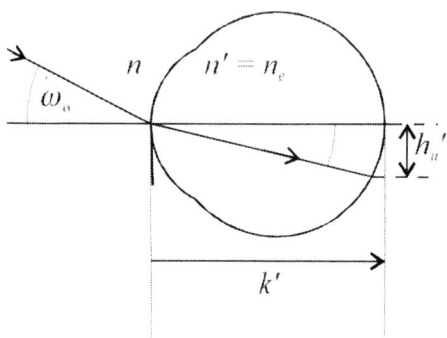

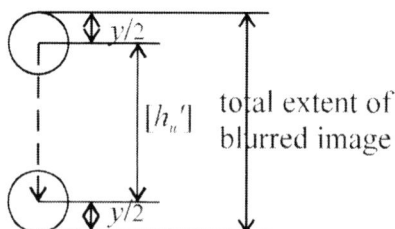

$$\overline{K}' = K + F_e$$
$$= -6 + 60 = +54D$$

$$h_u' = -\frac{1}{\overline{K}'}\tan\omega_o$$

$$= -\frac{1}{54}\tan 4° = -1.295mm$$

$$y = p\left[\frac{K}{\overline{K}'}\right]$$

$$y = 4\left[\frac{-6}{54}\right] = -0.\dot{4}mm$$

∴ the total extent of the blurred image

$$[h_u'] + y = -1.295 + (-0.\dot{4}) = -1.739mm$$

15. A thin +5D lens is used to correct an axially hypermetropic eye at 14mm from the reduced surface. A distant object subtending 3° is viewed through the lens. Find the ocular refraction, the axial length of the eye and the retinal image size in the uncorrected and corrected eye.

$$K = \frac{F}{1-dF} = \frac{5}{1-0.014 \times 5}$$
$$= +5.38D$$

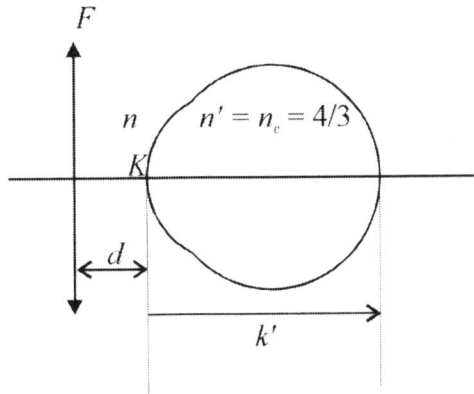

$$\overline{K}' = K + F_e = 5.38 + 60$$
$$= 65.38D$$

$$k' = \frac{n_e}{\overline{K}'} = \frac{4/3}{65.38}$$
$$= +20.394mm$$

$$h_u' = -\frac{1}{\overline{K}'}\tan\omega_o = -\frac{1}{65.38}\tan 3° = -0.802mm$$

$$h_c' = -f'\tan w_o \frac{K}{\overline{K}'} = -200\tan 3° \times \frac{5.376}{65.376} = -0.863mm$$

16. [a] Define the blurred retinal image size.
[Remember to include diagrams]
[b] An uncorrected axial myope views a distant object subtending 5Δ. The spectacle correction is –5.00DS at 13mm and the pupil diameter is 4mm.
Calculate [i] the size of the retinal blur disc and [ii] the total extent of the retina stimulated.

[a] Blurred retinal image size is the distance on the retina between the points where the chief rays from the top and the bottom of the object intersect the retina.

The diagram suitable to accompany this definition is Fig.2.14(a) from ITVO.

[b] [i]

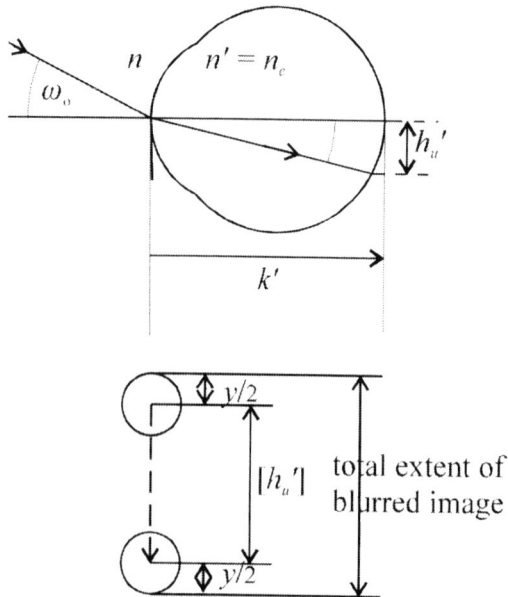

$$K = \frac{F}{(1 - dF)} = \frac{-5}{(1 - \{0.013 \times -5\})}$$

$$K = -4.69D$$

$$\overline{K}' = K + F_e = -4.69 + 60 = +55.31D$$

Blur disc diameter $= y = p\left[\dfrac{F_e}{\overline{K}'} - 1\right]$

[where p = pupil diameter]

[ii] Total extent of retina stimulated $= h_u' + y$

To find h_u', use $h_u' = -\frac{3}{4}k' \cdot \tan\omega_o$.

$$k' = \frac{n'}{\overline{K}'} = \frac{\frac{4}{3}}{55.31} = 0.024107m = 24.107mm$$

$$\tan\omega_o = \frac{5}{100}$$

$$\therefore h_u' = -\frac{3}{4} \times 24.107 \times \frac{5}{100} = -0.904mm$$

$\therefore$ Total extent of retina stimulated $= 0.904 + 0.339 = \underline{1.243mm}$

17. An uncorrected axial hypermetrope of ocular refraction $+7.00D$ and pupil diameter of $3mm$, views a distant object subtending $2.5'$.

Find [i] the retinal image size in the unaided eye [ii] full extent of image on retina [iii] the spectacle R_x if this eye is now corrected by a thin lens at $12mm$ vertex distance.

[Assume that the eye is unaccommodated at all times].

[i] $\overline{K}' = K + F_e = +7 + 60 = +67D$

$$\therefore k' = \frac{4/3}{67} = 0.019900m = 19.900mm$$

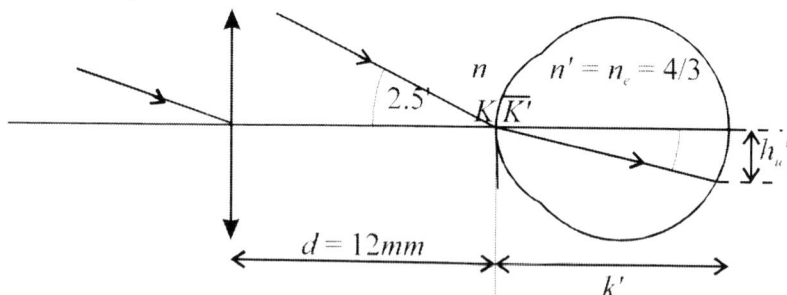

$h_u' = -\tfrac{3}{4} \cdot k' \cdot \tan \omega$

$h_u' = -0.75 \times 19.9 \times \tan 2.5'$

$\underline{h_u' = -0.01085mm}$

[ii] $y = p\left[\dfrac{F_e}{\overline{K}'} - 1\right] \therefore y = 3\left[\dfrac{60}{67} - 1\right] = -0.313mm$ Also draw

Fig.2.23(b)ITVO.

Total extent of retina stimulated

$h_u' + y = 0.01085 + 0.313 = \underline{0.324mm}$

[iii] $F = \dfrac{K}{(1+dK)} = \dfrac{7}{(1+0.012 \times 7)} = \underline{+6.46DS}$

20

18. A hypermetropic eye has $K = +9.09D$ and correcting lens $F = +8.00D$. Find the vertex distance and spectacle magnification.

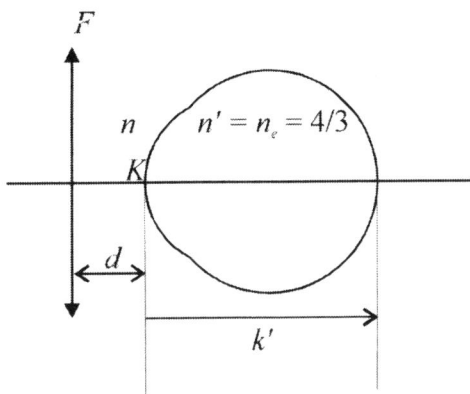

$$K = \frac{F}{1 - dF}$$

$$9.09 = \frac{8}{1 - d8}$$

$$\therefore 9.09 - 72.72d = 8$$

$$\therefore 72.72d = 1.09$$

$$d = \underline{0.015m}$$

For a thin lens with a reduced eye

$$SM = \frac{1}{1 - dF} = \frac{1}{1 - 0.015 \times 8} = \underline{1.136}$$

or

$$SM = \frac{K}{F} = \frac{9.09}{8} = 1.136$$

19. A refractively ametropic eye is corrected by $-9.00D$ placed $15mm$ from the reduced surface. It views a distant object subtending $3°$. Calculate the ocular refraction, the spectacle magnification, the uncorrected retinal image size and the corrected retinal image size.

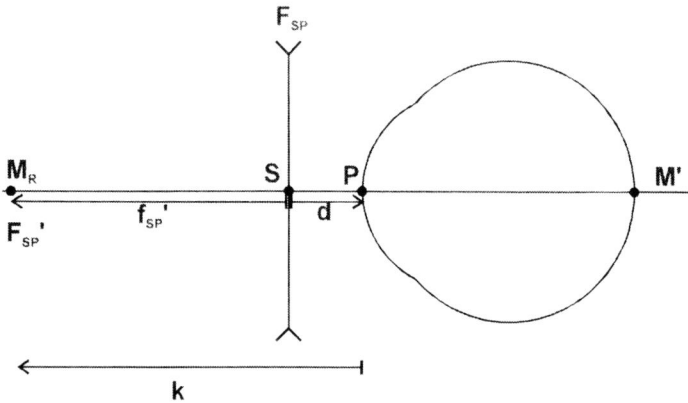

$$F_{SP} = -9.00D \quad \therefore \, f_{SP}{'} = \frac{1}{-9} = -0.\dot{1}m$$

$$d = 15mm \quad \therefore \, k = -0.\dot{1} - 0.015 = -0.126\dot{1}m = 126.111mm$$

$$K = \frac{1}{-0.126\dot{1}} = -7.93D$$

$$SM = \frac{K}{F_{SP}} = \frac{-7.93}{-9} = 0.881$$

Refractively ametropic eye so $k{'} = +0.022222m$ and $\overline{K}{'} = +60.00D$
$\omega = 3°$

Uncorrected retinal image size

$$h_u' = -\frac{1}{K'}\tan\omega_o = -\frac{(\tan 3°)}{60} = -0.000873m = -0.873mm$$

Corrected retinal image size

$$h_c' = h_u' \times SM = -0.873 \times 0.881 = -0.769mm$$

20. Use the diagram of the simplified schematic eye to calculate the retinal image size of a distant object subtending 5°

$$h_u' = -\frac{1}{K'}\tan\omega_0$$

$$h_u' = -\frac{1}{59.74}\tan 5°$$

$$h_u' = -1.464mm$$

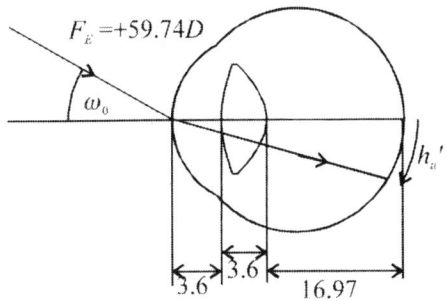

Uncorrected

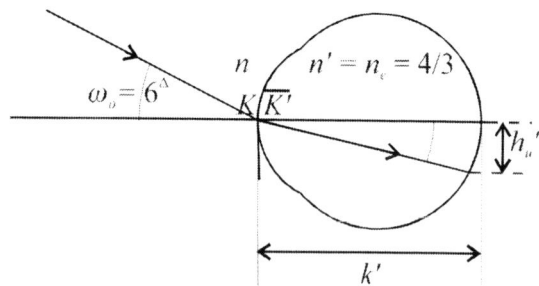

Corrected eye

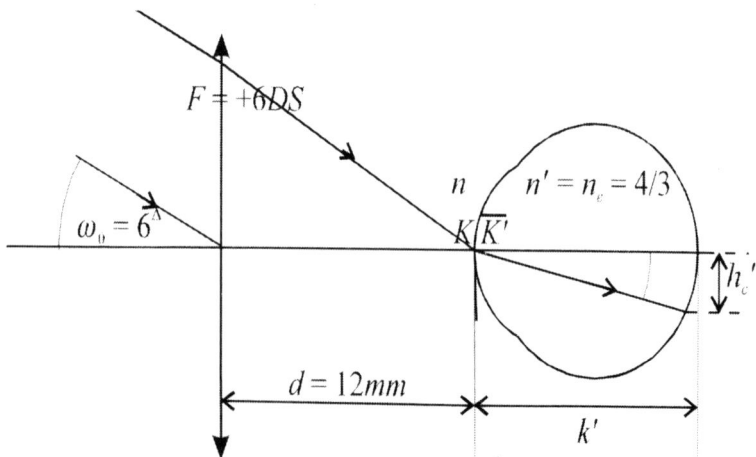

24

[i] [a] $K = \dfrac{F}{(1-dF)} = \dfrac{+6}{1-(0.012\times6)} = \underline{+6.47D}$

[b] $F_e = +60DS$ since ametropia is axial

$$\overline{K}' = K + F_e = +6.47 + 60 = +66.47D$$

$$k' = \frac{n'}{\overline{K}'} = \frac{4/3}{66.47} = +0.020059m = \underline{20.059mm}$$

[c] $h_c' = -f' \cdot \tan w_0 \cdot \dfrac{K}{\overline{K}'} = -\dfrac{1000}{+6} \times 0.06 \times \dfrac{6.47}{66.47} = \underline{-0.973mm}$

[d] $h_u' = -\dfrac{k'}{n} \cdot \tan w_0 = -\dfrac{20.059}{4/3} \times 0.06 = \underline{-0.903mm}$

[e] S.M. $= \dfrac{h_c'}{h_u'} = \dfrac{K}{F} = \dfrac{1}{1-dF} = \underline{1.078}$

[ii] Axial myope $-5.00DS$ @ $12mm$

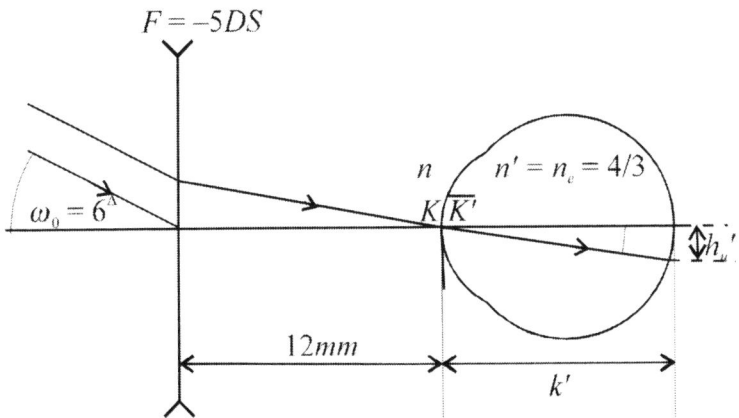

[a]

$$K = \frac{F}{(1 - dF)}$$

$$= \frac{-5}{(1 - 0.012 \times -5)}$$

$$= \underline{-4.72D}$$

[b] $\overline{K}' = K + F_e = -4.72 + 60 = +55.28D$

$$k' = \frac{n'}{\overline{K}'} = \frac{4/3}{55.28} = \underline{24.120mm}$$

[c] $h_c' = -f' \cdot \tan w_0 \cdot \frac{K}{\overline{K}'} = \frac{-1000}{-5} \times 0.06 \times \frac{-4.72}{+55.28} = \underline{-1.025mm}$

[d] $h_u' = -\frac{k'}{n_e'} \cdot \tan w_0 = -\frac{24.120}{4/3} \times 0.06 = \underline{-1.085mm}$

[e] S.M. $= \frac{h_c'}{h_u'} = \frac{K}{F} = \underline{0.944}$

---

22. [a] An eye with an ocular refraction of +7.50D is corrected by a thin lens at 13mm from the reduced surface. Calculate spectacle power and spectacle magnification.

[b] An uncorrected axial myope, ocular refraction −5.00D, views a distant object subtending 5^Δ. Calculate the retinal image size.

[c] What is the spectacle correction in [b] if the thin lens is 11mm from the reduced surface?

[d] Calculate the retinal image size in the corrected eye for [b]

[e] What would be the retinal image size in [b] if a contact lens was worn?

---

[a] $F = \dfrac{K}{(1+dK)} = \dfrac{7.50}{(1+0.013\times7.50)} = \underline{+6.83D}$

$\text{S.M.} = \dfrac{K}{F} = \dfrac{+7.50}{+6.83} = \underline{1.098}$

[b]
$K = -5D$
$F_e = +60DS$

$\overline{K}' = K + F_e = +55DS$

$k' = \dfrac{n'}{\overline{K}'} = 24.242mm.$

$h_u' = -\tfrac{3}{4}k'\tan w_0$

$h_u' = -\tfrac{3}{4}\times24.242\times\dfrac{5}{100} = \underline{0.909mm}$

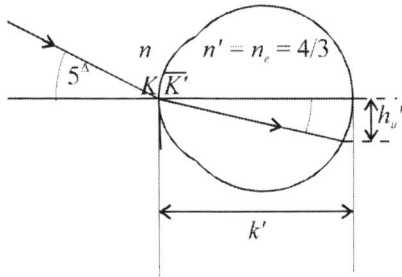

27

[c] $K = -5D$ $\quad$ $F = \dfrac{K}{1+dK} = \dfrac{-5}{(1+0.011\times -5)} = \underline{-5.29DS}$

[d] $h_u' = -\dfrac{k'}{n'}\cdot \tan\omega_0 = \underline{0.909mm}$

$$h_c' = S.M.\times h_u' = \dfrac{K}{F_v'}\times h_u' = \dfrac{-5.00}{-5.29}\times 0.909 = \underline{0.859mm}$$

[e] When a contact lens is worn, there is no vertex distance, $\therefore h_c' = h_u'$

$\therefore S.M. = 1$ and $h_c' = h_u' = \underline{0.909mm}$

23. A refractively myopic eye whose ocular refraction is –12.50D is corrected by a thin lens at 15mm.
Find [a] power of spectacle lens
[b] spectacle magnification
[c] retinal image sizes for a distant object subtending 4^{Δ}, corrected and uncorrected.
[d] R.S.M.

[a] $K = -12.50DS$ $d = 15mm.$

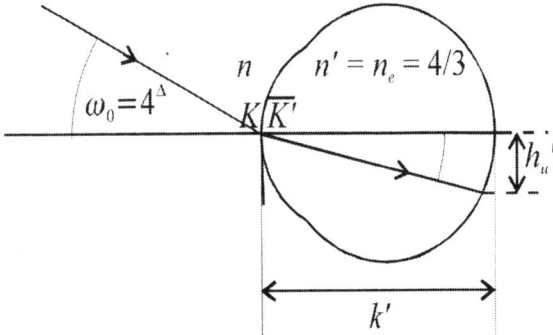

$$F = \frac{K}{1+dK} = \frac{-12.50}{1+(0.015 \times -12.50)}$$
$$= -15.38DS$$

[b] $S.M. = \frac{K}{F_v{}'} = \frac{-12.50}{-15.38} = 0.813$$

[c]

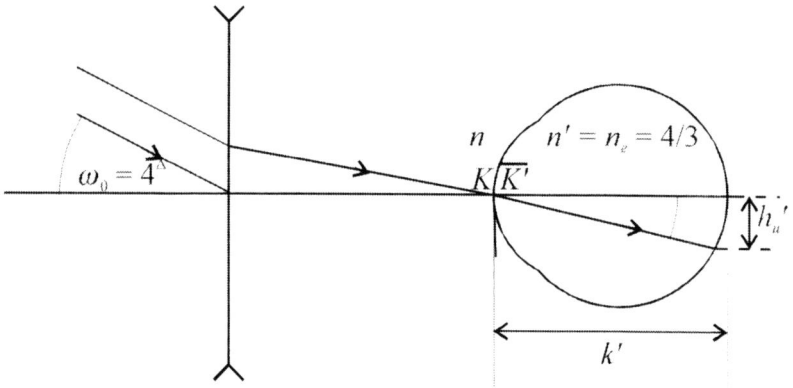

$$\overline{K}' = +60D$$

$$h_u' = -\frac{k'}{n'} \cdot \tan w_0$$

$$= -\frac{22.22}{4/3} \times 0.04$$

$$= \underline{0.667mm}$$

$$h_c' = S.M. \times h_u' = 0.813 \times 0.667 = \underline{0.542mm}$$

[e] RSM = 1 since it applies only to <u>axial</u> ametropia. In this case, the ametropia is refractive, and so RSM has no effect.

---

24. A refractively hypermetropic eye focuses a 20*mm* high object 50*cm* from the eye [a] with the +4.00*D* thin correcting lens at 15*mm* from the reduced surface and [b] without the correction. Find the retinal image sizes and ocular accommodation in both cases.

---

[a] $K = \dfrac{F}{1-dF} = \dfrac{+4}{1-0.015\times4} = +4.26D$

$\overline{K}' = +60D$

$\therefore h_c' = -f'\tan\omega_o \dfrac{K}{\overline{K}'} = -250\times\dfrac{0.020}{0.50}\times\dfrac{4.26}{60} = -0.71mm$

$L_{eye} = -\dfrac{1}{-50} = +2D$
$\therefore A_{oc} = K - L_{eye} = 4.26 - 2 = +2.26D$

[b] Because the hypermetropia is refractive, $k' = +22.222mm$. n_e is assumed to be 4/3.

$h_u' = -\dfrac{k'}{n_e}\tan w_o = -\dfrac{22.222}{^4\!/_3}\times\dfrac{0.020}{0.50} = -0.667mm$

Uncorrected $L = -2D$ $\therefore A_{oc} = 4.26 - (-2) = +6.26D$

A thin lens has a plane back surface and a front surface with principal powers +2.50D horizontally and +3.50D vertically. An axial object point 0.4m to the left of the lens images the horizontal line focus on a screen to the right of the lens. Find the position of the screen and the distance the object must be moved to image the vertical line focus on the screen.

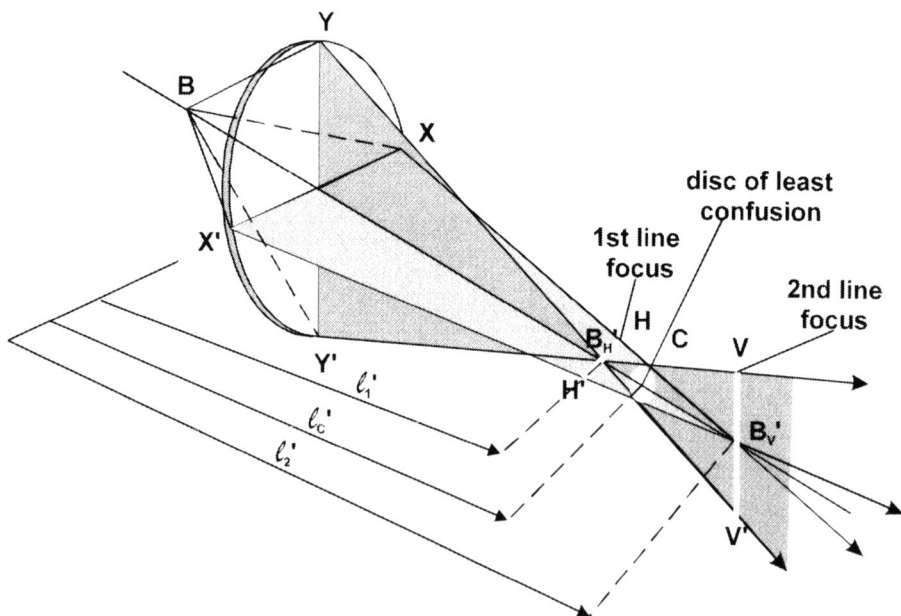

$F' = +3.50D$ $L = -2.50D$

$L' = F + L$ $\therefore L' = +3.5 + [-2.5] = +1D \quad l' = 1.0m$

i.e. screen is 1m to the right of the lens.

In order to bring the vertical line focus on to the screen L' will remain as $+1D$ with $F = +2.5D$

From $L = L' - F$ we get $L = +1 - [+2.5] = -1.5D$ $l = -0.66m$, therefore the image must be moved from -1.0 to $-0.66m$ i.e. $33cm$ to the right of its original position.

An unaccommodated eye of standard length has an ocular ametropia of $+2.00/+3.00 \times 60$. It views a point object at $1m$ from the reduced surface. If the pupil diameter is $4mm$ find the positions of the line foci formed by the eye and the dimensions of the blurred patch on the retina.

What lens at a distance of $15mm$ from the reduced surface would correct this eye for distance vision?

Axis 60

$k' = +22.222mm$

So $\overline{K}' = +60.00D$

$K = +5.00D \times 60$

$F_e = \overline{K}' - K = 60 - 5$
$= +55.00D \times 60$
$\ell = -1m$ So $L = -1.00D$
$L' = L + F_e = -1 + 55$
$= +54.00D \times 60$

$\ell' = \dfrac{n'}{L'} = \dfrac{\left(1000 \times \frac{4}{3}\right)}{54}$
$= +24.691mm$

    The 60 line image is at $+24.691mm$

Axis 150

$\overline{K}' = +60.00D$

$K = +2.00D \times 150$

$F_e = 60 - 2$
$= +58.00D \times 150$
$L = -1.00D$
$L' = -1 + 58$
$= +57.00D \times 150$

$\ell' = \dfrac{\left(1000 \times \frac{4}{3}\right)}{57}$
$= +23.392mm$

    The 150 line image is at $+23.392mm$

The positions of the line images

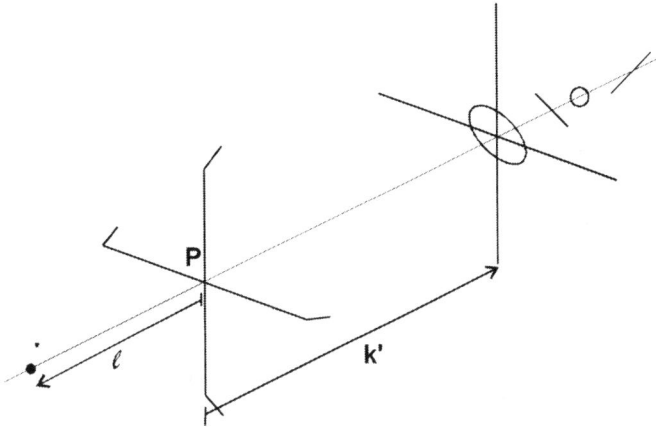

$p = 4mm$

$$y = \frac{p(K'-L')}{K'}$$

$$= \frac{4(60-54)}{60} = 0.400mm$$

$p = 4mm$

$$y = \frac{4(60-57)}{60} = 0.200mm$$

The retinal blur is an ellipse, 0.400*mm* along 150 and 0.200*mm* along 60

Hyperopic corrected eye

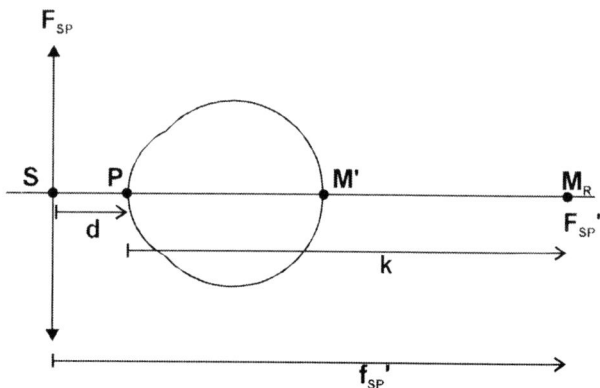

$K = +5.00D \times 60$	$K = +2.00D \times 150$
$k = +20.00cm$	$k = +50.00cm$
$d = 15mm = 1.5cm$	$d = 1.5cm$
$f_{SP}' = +21.5cm$	$f_{SP}' = +51.5cm$
$F_{SP} = +4.65D \times 60$	$F_{SP} = +1.94D \times 150$

The spectacle correction is $+1.94D/+2.71D \times 60$

27. A reduced eye with refractive ametropia has an ocular refraction of $-3.00DS/-3.00DC \times 180$.
[a] Calculate the spectacle R_x at a vertex distance of $12mm$, and state the type of astigmatism.
[b] Calculate the focal line positions when the unaided eye views a point object $\frac{1}{3}m$ from the eye. Which focal line is nearest to the retina?
[c] Calculate the principal radii of curvature of the reduced surface. Is this astigmatism 'with' or 'against' the rule?
[d] Find the size of the blur ellipse on the retina when viewing a distant object uncorrected, if the pupil size is $4.5mm$.

[a] $K = -3.00DS/-3.00DC \times 180$;

$d = 12mm$

$\therefore K$ along 90
   $= -6.00D$
and
K along 180
   $= -3.00D$

$F = \dfrac{K}{(1+dK)}$

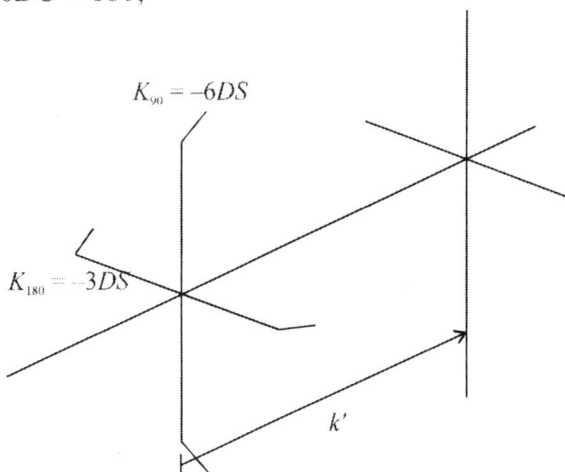

$K_{90} = -6DS$

$K_{180} = -3DS$

k'

Along 90° meridian

$\therefore F_{90} = \dfrac{-6}{1+(0.012 \times -6)}$

$= -6.47DS$

Along 180° meridian

$\therefore F_{180} = \dfrac{-3}{1+(0.012 \times -3)}$

$= -3.11DS$

$\therefore$ Spectacle $R_x = -3.11DS/-3.36DC \times 180$

Type of astigmatism: Compound Myopic Astigmatism.

[b] $\overline{K}' = +60D$ since ametropia is refractive

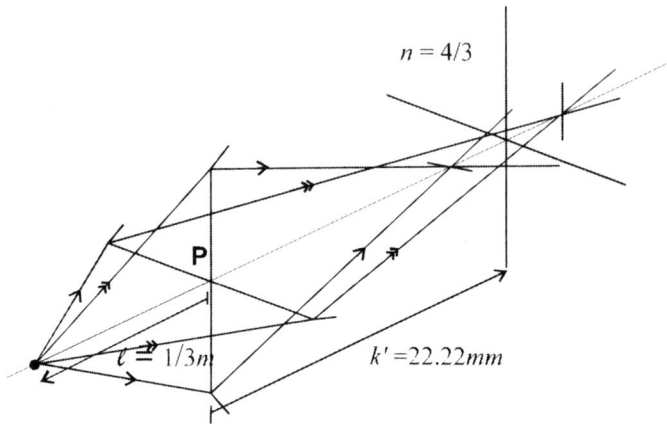

$$F_e = \overline{K}' - K$$

Along 90° meridian

$$F_e = +60 - (-5.60)$$
$$F_e = +65.60DS$$
$$\overline{L} = -3.00D$$
$$\overline{L}' = L + F_e$$
$$\therefore \overline{L}' = -3.00 + 65.60 = 62.60D$$
$$\therefore \ell' = \frac{4/3}{62.60} = 21.299mm.$$
[*Horiz.line*]

Along 180° meridian

$$F_e = +60 - (-2.90)$$
$$F_e = +62.90DS$$
$$\overline{L} = -3.00D$$
$$\overline{L}' = L + F_e$$
$$\therefore \overline{L}' = -3.00 + 62.90 = 59.90D$$
$$\therefore \ell' = \frac{4/3}{59.90} = 22.259mm.$$
[*Vert.line*]

Since the length of the reduced eye in refractive ametropia is 22.22*mm*, the vertical line focus will be formed nearest to the retina −0.039*mm* behind the retina.

[c] Using $F = \dfrac{(n'-n)}{r}$ $\therefore r_c = \dfrac{n'-n}{F_e}$

Along 90° meridian

$$r_c = \frac{(\tfrac{4}{3}-1)}{+65.6}$$
$$r_c = 0.005081m = 5.081mm$$

Along 180° meridian

$$r_c = \frac{(\tfrac{4}{3}-1)}{+62.9}$$
$$r_c = 0.005299m = 5.299mm$$

∴ Radius along 90° = 5.081*mm* and radius along 180° = 5.299*mm*

Since the radius is steeper in the vertical meridian, this astigmatism is 'with' the rule.

[d]

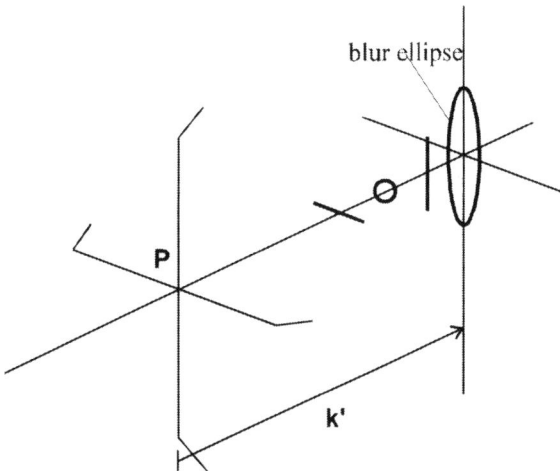

Pupil size $p = 4.5mm$ diameter

Retinal image $y = p\left[\dfrac{K}{K'}\right]$

Horizontal retinal image size $\qquad$ Vertical retinal image size

$$y_V = 4.5\left[\dfrac{-6.0}{60}\right] = 0.450mm \qquad y_H = 4.5\left[\dfrac{-3.0}{60}\right] = 0.225mm$$

$\therefore$ The blur ellipse is a vertical ellipse 0.450mm high and 0.225mm wide

28. A reduced eye has principal powers $F_{e,45} = +63D$ and $F_{e,135} = +65D$, the axial length being $21.505mm$ and $n_e = 1.3333$. For a distant axial object point, find the position of the line foci 'relative to the retina'.

The dioptric value of the axial length is

$$\overline{K}' = \frac{n_e}{k'} = \frac{1.3333}{0.021505} = +62.00D$$

Therefore the 45° meridian is too strong by $1.00D$ and will form a line focus at 135° and $-1.00D$ in front of the retina. The 135° meridian is too powerful by $3.00D$ and will consequently form a line focus at 45° and $-3.00D$ in front of the retina.

This can be verified by putting $L = 0$ in each meridian giving:

$$\overline{L}_{45}' = F_{e,45} = +63D \text{ and } \overline{L}_{135}' = F_{e,135} = +65D$$

which shows the positions of the line foci to be in front of the retina since the dioptric length of the eye is $+62.00D$.

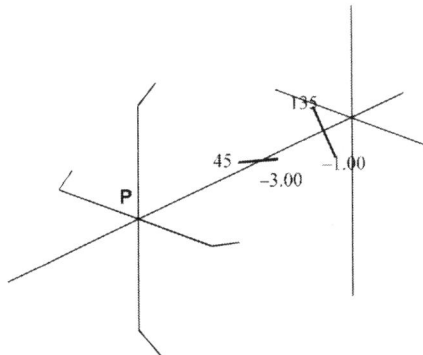

$F = +9DS$

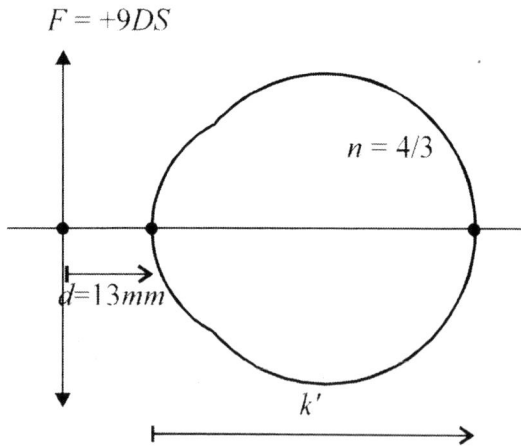

$n = 4/3$

$d = 13mm$

k'

[a] For a thin lens, $S.M. = \dfrac{1}{(1-dF)} = \dfrac{1}{(1-0.013 \times 9)} = \underline{1.133}$

[b] For a thick lens, $S.M. = \dfrac{1}{(1-dF_v')} \times \dfrac{1}{(1-\bar{t}F_1)}$

$F_v' = +9.00DS$; $F_2 = -6.00DS$; $t = 7mm$; $n_g = 1.51$

To find F_1 use either $F_1 = \dfrac{F_v{'} - F_2}{1 + \bar{t}\left(F_v{'} - F_2\right)}$ or trace rays through

the lens from R → L using step-back

$L_1 = 0.00D$; $L_2{'} = F_v{'} = +9.00D$; $\bar{L}_2 = L_2{'} - F_2 = +15.00D$;

$\dfrac{t}{n} = \dfrac{7}{1.51} = 4.636mm$.

$\bar{L}_1{'} = \dfrac{\bar{L}_2}{1 + \bar{t}\bar{L}_2}$

$\bar{L}_1{'} = \dfrac{+15.00}{1 + 0.00464 \times 15}$

$\bar{L}_1{'} = +14.02D = F_1$

So,

$S.M. = \dfrac{1}{\left(1 - \{0.013 \times 9\}\right)} \times \dfrac{1}{\left(1 - \{0.004636 \times 14.02\}\right)}$

$= 1.133 \times 1.0695 = \underline{1.211}$

[c] The more accurate value, obtained when considering a thick lens, shows a value greater than that determined assuming a thin lens correction. From the results in [a] and [b] it can be seen that, if the thickness of a lens is not taken into account, then an artificially low value for *S.M.* is obtained. This is significant since subjects can detect a change in retinal image size of as little as 0.25%.

In the example, *S.M.* with thin lens is 13.25% increase
and *S.M.* with thick lens is 21.1% increase.

30. A patient has axial myopia - R. $-1.50DS$ L. $-10.50DS$
If a distant object subtends $2°$, calculate
  [a] uncorrected image size
  [b] image size when corrected by thin spectacle lenses at
     $13mm$
  [c] image size when corrected by thin contact lens
Repeat for a patient with refractive myopia,
R. $-1.50DS$ L. $-10.50DS$

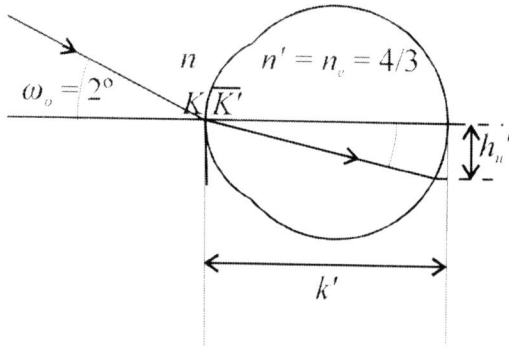

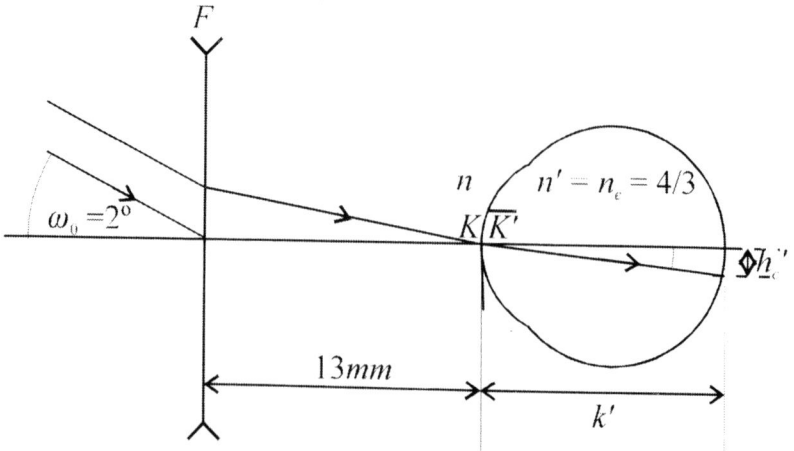

[a] Myopia is axial, $\therefore F_e = +60DS.$ $\overline{K}' = K + F_e$

$$\therefore \overline{K}_R' = -1.50 + 60 = +58.50D \qquad \therefore \overline{K}_L' = -10.50 + 60 = +49.50D$$

$$\therefore k_R' = \frac{n'}{\overline{K}_R'} = \frac{4/3}{+58.50} \qquad \therefore k_L' = \frac{n'}{\overline{K}_L'} = \frac{4/3}{+49.50}$$

$$\therefore k_R' = 22.792mm. \qquad \therefore k_L' = 26.936mm.$$

$$h_u' = -\tfrac{3}{4} \cdot k' \cdot \tan w$$

Right	Left
$h_u' = -\tfrac{3}{4} \times 22.792 \times \tan 2^\circ$	$h_u' = -\tfrac{3}{4} \times 26.936 \times \tan 2^\circ$
$\underline{h_u' = -0.597mm}$	$\underline{h_u' = -0.705mm}$

[b] $$F = \frac{K}{1 + dK}$$

Right	Left
$\therefore F = -1.53DS$	$F = -12.16DS$

$$S.M. = \frac{K}{F}$$

Right	Left
$\therefore S.M. = \dfrac{-1.50}{-1.53} = \underline{0.980}$	$\therefore S.M. = \dfrac{-10.50}{-12.16} = \underline{0.863}$

$$h_c' = S.M. \times h_u'$$

Right	Left
$\therefore h_c' = 0.980 \times -0.597$	$\therefore h_c' = 0.863 \times -0.705$
$\underline{h_c' = -0.585mm}$	$\underline{h_c' = -0.608mm}$

[c] With contact lenses, $S.M. = 1$.

$$\therefore h_c' = -0.597mm \qquad\qquad \text{and } h_c' = -0.705mm$$

If the myopia is refractive: $\qquad \overline{K}' = +60DS$

$$F_c = \overline{K}' - K \qquad\qquad k' = +22.22mm$$

Right   Left

$$\therefore F_c = +60 - (-1.50) \qquad\qquad \therefore F_c = +60 - (-10.50)$$
$$= +61.50D \qquad\qquad\qquad = +70.50D$$

[a]

$$h_u' = -\tfrac{3}{4} \times 22.22 \times \tan 2°$$
$$h_u' = -0.582mm$$

for both R. & L. since the axial lengths are equal.

[b] $S.M. = \dfrac{K}{F} \qquad \therefore S.M_R = 0.980 \text{ and } S.M_L = 0.863$ as previously calculated.

$$h_c' = S.M. \times h_u'$$

$$\therefore h_c' = 0.980 \times -0.582 \qquad\qquad h_c' = 0.863 \times -0.58$$
$$= -0.570mm \qquad\qquad\qquad = -0.502mm$$

[c] With contact lenses, $S.M. = 1 \qquad \therefore h_c' = -0.582mm$ R & L

From the results obtained, for axial myopia, the difference in retinal image sizes is less with spectacles than with contact lenses. However, when the error is refractive, a better result is obtained with contact lenses, there being greater discrepancy in retinal image sizes with the spectacle correction.

> **31.** [a] What effects will be noticed by a patient who becomes bilaterally aphakic?
> [b] An axial myope corrected by $-3.00DS$ @ 15mm has a corneal radius of 7.55mm. This eye becomes aphakic. Determine the power of the spectacle lens for a vertex distance of 15mm.

[a] The action of removing the crystalline lens has three immediate effects on a patient.

- It renders them highly hypermetropic, usually in the region of $+12DS$, and hence a high positive correcting lens is needed.
- without the lens there is no accommodative ability
- the main U-V protection for the retina is absent.

Although a large proportion of patients are now corrected with an intraocular implant following lens removal, if is not the case, then, when corrected with the appropriate spectacle lens, the patient will notice/experience;

- objects appearing to be out of proportion due to larger retinal image size than previously.
- misjudging distances due to the enlarged retinal image size.
- no clear near vision possible without the addition of reading correction in the order of +3 to +3.50DS on top of the distance R_x.
- distortion away from the centres of the lenses
- reduced field of view
- prismatic effects away from the optical centres
- photophobia.

Each of these points should be briefly discussed, together with the possible solutions to the problems.

[b] see Fig.2.3 ITVO

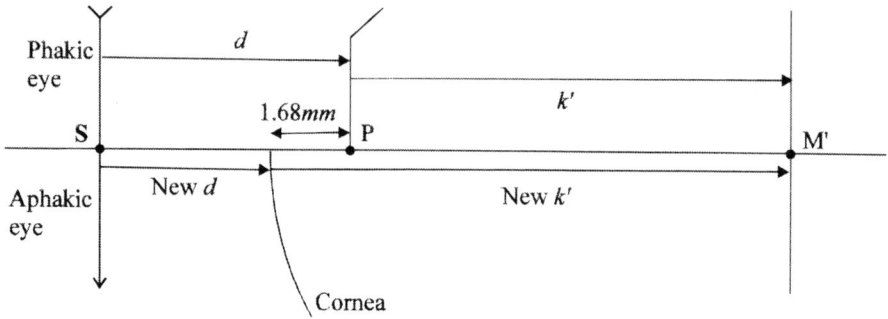

Phakic eye: $K = -3.00DS; \quad \overline{K}' = 60 - 3 = +57D$

$$\therefore k' = \frac{\tfrac{4}{3}}{57} = 23.392mm$$

Aphakic eye: New axial length is $1.68mm$ longer

$$\therefore k_c' = 25.072mm$$

$$\overline{K}' = \frac{n'}{k'} = \frac{\tfrac{4}{3}}{0.025072} = +53.18D$$

$r_c = 7.55mm$

$$F_e = \frac{1000(n-1)}{r_c}$$

$$F_e = \frac{333.3}{7.55} = +44.15DS$$

New $K - F_e = +53.18 - 44.15 = +9.03D$

$$k = \frac{1000}{K} = 110.743mm$$

New $d = 15 - 1.68 = 13.32mm$

$$F = \frac{K}{(1 + dK)} \quad \therefore F = \frac{9.03}{1 + 0.01332 \times 9.03} = +8.06DS$$

∴ Power of the spectacle lens $= +8.06DS$

32.	An eye with axial length 24.464mm and refractive index 1.3333 has reduced surface powers of +57.00D and +63.00D horizontally and vertically, respectively. Find the ocular refractions and the principal powers of the thin correcting lens at 15mm.

The dioptric length of the eye is:

$$\overline{K}' = \frac{n_e}{k'} = \frac{1.3333}{0.024464} = +54.50D.$$

The principal powers of the reduced surface are

$$F_{e,180} = +57.00D \qquad F_{e,90} = +63.00D$$

so the ocular refractions in the principal meridians are

$$K_{180} = \overline{K}' - F_{e,180} = (+54.50) - (+57.00) = -2.50D$$
$$K_{90} = \overline{K}' - F_{e,90} = (+54.50) - (+63.00) = -8.50D$$

Therefore stepping back through the vertex distance d

$$F_{180} = \frac{K_{180}}{1 + dK_{180}} = \frac{-2.50}{1 + 0.015 \times -2.50} = -2.60D$$

$$F_{90} = \frac{K_{90}}{1 + dK_{90}} = \frac{-8.50}{1 + 0.015 \times -8.50} = -9.74D$$

$$\therefore R_x = -2.60DS/-7.14DC \times 180$$

33. An eye is corrected by a thin lens with power +4.00DS/+3.00DC × 45 at 10*mm*. If the refractive index of the eye is 1.3333 and the reduced surface power is +61.00*D* along 135°, find the axial length of the eye and the eye's power along 45°.

First find the powers along the principal meridians of the lens:

$$F_{45} = +4.00D \qquad F_{135} = +7.00D$$

The eye's power along 135° is known so, if we find the ocular refraction K_{135}, we will be able to find the dioptric length of the eye from the equation $\overline{K}' = K + F_e$ applied to the meridian.

$$K_{135} = \frac{F_{135}}{1 - dF_{135}} = \frac{+7.00}{1 - 0.010 \times 7.00} = +7.53D$$

and then $\overline{K}' = K_{135} + F_{e,135} = (+7.53) + (+61.00) = +68.53D$

from which $k' = \dfrac{n_e}{\overline{K}'} = \dfrac{1.3333}{68.53} = +0.019456m = +19.456mm$

We must now find $F_{e,45}$ using the equation $F_e = \overline{K}' - K$:

$$F_{e,45} = \overline{K}' - K_{45} = \overline{K}' - \frac{F_{45}}{1 - dF_{45}}$$

$$F_{e,45} = (+68.53) - \frac{+4.00}{1 - 0.010 \times +4.00} = +64.36D.$$

34. An eye can just read the *3m* letters on a test chart at *6m*. What is the Snellen acuity ? What is the decimal acuity ?

If the test chart is moved to a distance of 24m from the subject, what is the size and height of the letters that can be just distinguished ? How would the Snellen acuity be recorded now ?

If the pupil diameter is *4mm*, give an estimate of the amount of ametropia that this eye might have.

Testing distance is *6m* and the Best Line is *3m* so the Snellen acuity is 6/3

Converting this to a decimal gives the decimal acuity of 2.0.

Calculations of this type can either be done by using similar triangles as shown in the unit or by finding the MAR as shown in Tunnacliffe's Introduction to Visual Optics.

By MAR

6/3 is the same as 1/0.50 So the MAR is 0.50'

At 24m the letter size that would be read is given by $24 \times 0.50 = 12m$

So the Best Line is the *12m* line and the letter height on this line is $12000 \times \tan 5'$

$= 17.45mm$

OR by similar triangles

Height of *3m* letter is $3000 \times \tan 5' = 4.36mm$

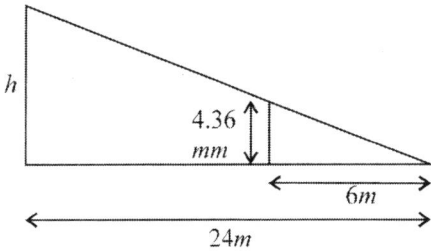

To find the height read at
24m
h = 24 × 4.36/6
= 17.45mm

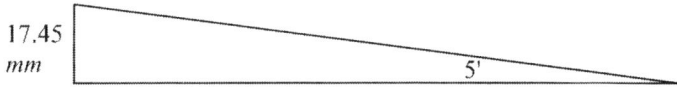

This letter subtends 5'
at 17.45/tan 5'
= 12000mm
= 12m

So the letter size read at 24m is the 12m line.

Snellen acuity is now 24/12

To estimate ametropia

$D = 4pK$ where D is best line

$K = D/4p$

$D = 12m$ and $p = 4mm$

So $K = 12/(4 \times 4) = 0.75D$

35. [a] A subject can read 2.5*mm* high print at a distance of 50*cm*. What would be their acuity at 6*m*?

[b] A subject has a VA of 4/12. Calculate the height of the letters that can be read at 35*cm*.

[a]

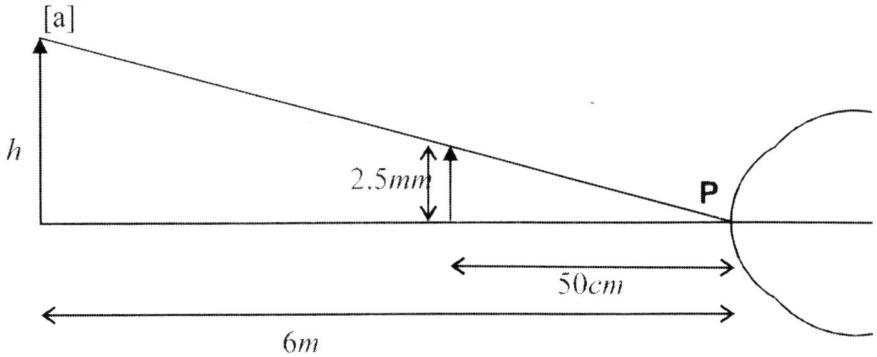

Find the letter height at 6*m* by similar triangles

From the above diagram, $\dfrac{h}{6000} = \dfrac{2.5}{500}$ $\therefore h = 30mm$.

The letter 30*mm* high will thus subtend 5′ at *x* metres.
   [think about the definition of Snellen Acuity]

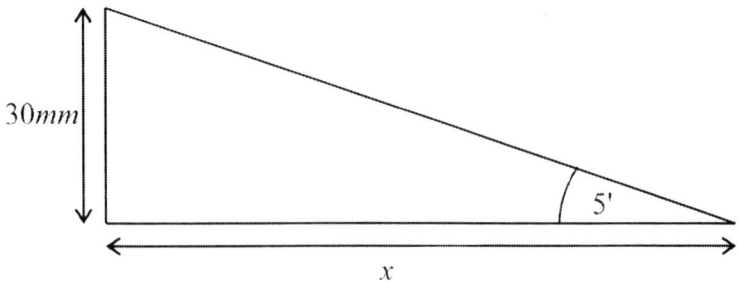

$$\therefore x = \frac{30}{\tan 5'} = 20626mm$$
$$\therefore \underline{x = 20.63m}$$

Hence, the patient would be able to easily read the 6/24 line, and probably a little more, since the accurate VA is 6/20.6

[b] Letter height = testing distance × tan 5′
$$= 4 \times \tan 5'$$
$$= 5.818mm$$

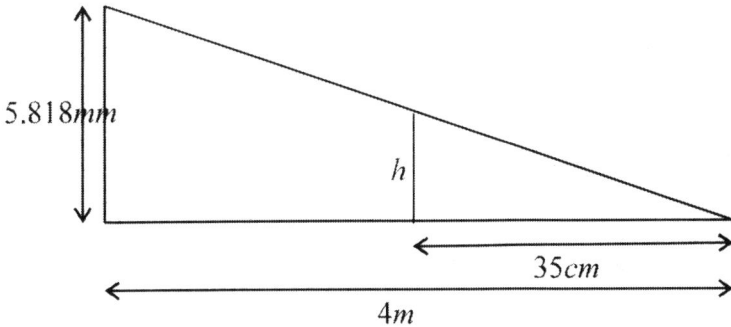

From similar triangles, $\dfrac{h}{350} = \dfrac{5.818}{4000} mm$

$$\therefore h = 5.818 \times \frac{350}{4000}$$
$$\therefore \underline{h = 0.510mm}$$

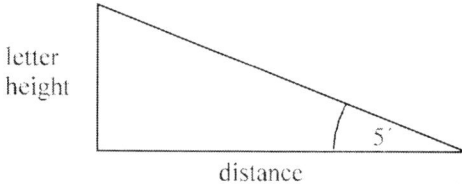

$$\text{distance} = \frac{\text{letter height}}{\tan 5'}$$

$$= \frac{17.46}{0.001454} = 12.008m \approx 12m$$

We can therefore write the acuity in Snellen notation as:

$$VA = \frac{\text{testing distance in metres}}{\text{distance at which the height of the letters on the best row is 5'}}$$

$$= \frac{3}{12}$$

This can be converted to the standard 6*m* designation i.e. 6/24 which in decimal notation is 0.25.

37. Calculate the Snellen acuity required to read N6 print at 30*cm*. Assume an x- height Times New Roman font to be 0.9375*mm* and that it has a 1:5 limb width to letter height ratio and the limb width is constant around the letter.

The letter will have a limb width of 0.9375/5 = 0.1875*mm*. At 30*cm* [300*mm*] this limb width subtends an angle ω given by:

$$\tan \omega = 0.1875/300 = 0.000625$$

from which ω = arctan 0.000625 = 0.035810° = 2.15′

Hence, the resolution acuity is $VA_{RES} = \dfrac{1}{\omega} = \dfrac{1}{2.15} = 0.465$

which converts to Snellen notation by multiplying $\dfrac{1}{2.15}$ by $\dfrac{6}{6}$ which gives 6/12.9.

Given the above a patient with 6/12 acuity should be able to read N6 print at 30*cm*.

38. A reduced eye has an axial length of $+22.60mm$ and a power of $+63.00D$. Calculate the power of the thin spectacle lens placed at $15mm$ required to correct this eye for distance vision. This eye views a $24m$ Snellen letter on a test chart at $6m$. Find the uncorrected and the corrected retinal image sizes.

If this eye has a pupil diameter of $4mm$, what would be the total retinal image size formed in the uncorrected eye ?

$k' = +22.60mm \quad \overline{K}' = n'/k' = (1000 \times 4/3)/22.60 = +59.00D$

$F_e = +63.00D \quad K = \overline{K}' - F_e = 59.00 - 63.00 = -4.00D$

$K = -4.00D \quad k = 100/-4.00 = -25.00cm$
$d = 15mm = 1.5cm$

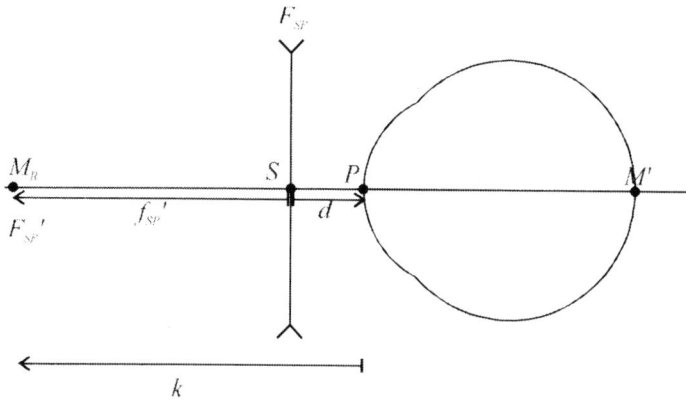

$f_{SP}' = -25.0 + 1.5 = -23.5cm$
So $F_{SP} = -4.26D$

Height of $24m$ letter is
$24000 \times \tan 5' = 34.91mm$
Tan $\omega_o = 34.91/6000$

$h_u' = -\left(\tan w_o / \overline{K}'\right)$
$= -1000 \times 34.91/6000)/59.00$
$= -0.099mm$

$h_c' = h_u' \times SM$

$SM = K/F_{SP} = -4.00/-4.26 = 0.939$
$h_c' = -0.099 \times 0.939 = -0.093mm$

Total retinal image size $= h_u' + y$

$6m$ can be considered as infinity so the relationship $y = pK/\overline{K}'$ can be used.

$y = 4 \times 4.00/59.00 = 0.271mm$

Total retinal image size $= 0.099 + 0.271 = 0.370mm$

39. A patient can read print of 1.75*mm* height at 30*cm*. What would be the VA at 5*m*?
A patient has a VA of 6/15. Calculate the height of letters that can be read at 50*cm*.

By similar triangles

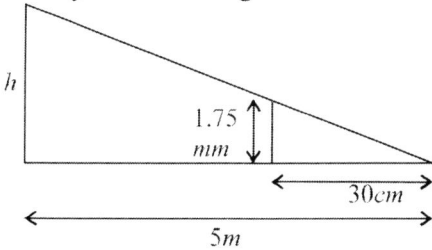

Letter height at 5*m*
= 5000 × 1.75/300
= 29.17*mm*

This letter subtends 5' at
29.17/tan 5'
= 20056*mm* = 20.056*m*
VA = 5/20

OR by MAR

Limb width = 1.75/5 = 0.35*mm*
So MAR = arctan 0.35/300 = 4'

Letter size at 5*m* = 5 × 4 = 20*m*

So the patient could read a 20*m* letter so the VA would be 5/20

By similar triangles
Height of 15*m* letter = 15000 × tan 5' = 21.82*mm*

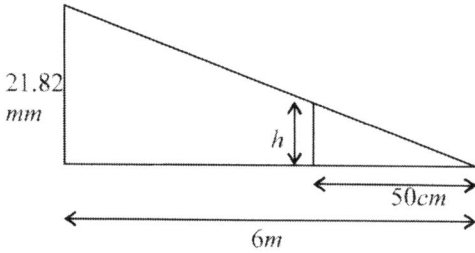

Height of letter that can be
read at 50*cm*
= 500 × 21.82/6000
= 1.82*mm*

21.82 *mm*

h

50*cm*

6*m*

OR by MAR

VA = 6/15 which is 1/2.5 So the MAR is 2.5'

The limb width at 50*cm* = 500 × tan 2.5' = 0.364*mm*

So the height of the letters is 5 × 0.364*mm* = 1.82*mm*

61

40. A patient is corrected for distance vision by the thin lens +8.50/−4.50 × 90 placed at 15mm from the reduced surface. If the axial length of the eye is +22.00*mm* calculate the ocular refraction and the radii of curvature of the reduced surface.

If this patient views a distant square object subtending 4Δ, find the size of the corrected retinal image.

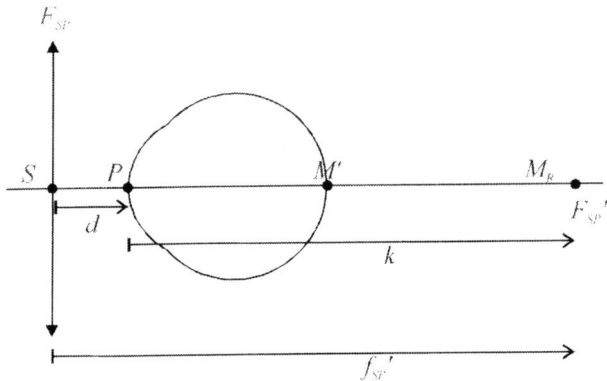

$$F_{SP} = +8.50/-4.50 \times 90 = +8.50 \times 180/+4.00 \times 90$$

Axis 180	**Axis 90**
$f_{SP}' = 100/8.5 = +11.76cm$	$f_{SP}' = 100/4 = +25cm$
$d = 15mm = 1.5cm$	$d = 1.5cm$
$k = +10.26cm$	$k = +23.50cm$
$K = 100/10.26 =$	$K = 100/23.50$
$+9.75D \times 180$	$= +4.26D \times 90$

Ocular refraction is $+9.75/-5.49 \times 90$

$k' = +22mm$

$\overline{K}' = n'/k' = (1000 \times 4/3)/22$
$= +60.61D$ $\qquad$ $\overline{K}' = +60.61D$

$F_e = \overline{K}' - K = 60.61 - 9.75$ $\qquad$ $F_e = 60.61 - 4.26$
$= +50.86D \times 180$ $\qquad$ $= +56.35D \times 90$

$r = (n' - n)/F_e$
$= (1000 \times (4/3 - 1))/50.86$ $\qquad$ $r = (1000 \times (4/3 - 1))/56.35$
$r = +6.55mm$ along 90 $\qquad$ $r = +5.92mm$ along 180

$h_c' = h_u' \times SM$ where $h_u' = -(tan\ w)/\overline{K}'$ and $SM = K/F_{SP}$

For both meridians $\omega = 4\Delta$ So tan $\omega = 4/100$
$h_u' = -(1000 \times 4/100)/60.61 = -0.66mm$

$SM = 9.75/8.5 = 1.147$ $\qquad$ $SM = 4.26/4 = 1.065$

$h_c' = -0.66 \times 1.147$ $\qquad$ $h_c' = -0.66 \times 1.065$
$= -0.757mm$ $\qquad$ $= -0.703mm$

Retinal image is $0.757mm$ high and $0.703mm$ wide.

41. **[a]** A refractive myope with ocular refraction of –5.00D wears his spectacle correction at 15*mm* from the reduced surface.
   [i] Find both the spectacle and ocular accommodation required to clearly observe an object 25*cm* from the lens.
   [ii] Calculate the retinal image size for an object 17.11*mm* high
   [HINT: remember that this is a <u>near</u> object and so S.M. cannot be used].
[b] Repeat [a] for a refractive hypermetrope of +5.00D.

[a] [i]

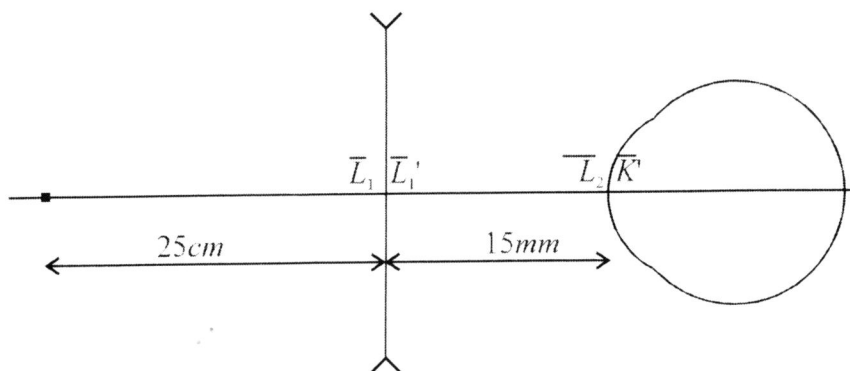

Myopia is refractive, $\therefore \overline{K}' = +60D$

$$F_v' = \frac{K}{(1+dK)}$$

$$F_v' = \frac{-5}{1+(0.015 \times -5)}$$

$$F_v' = -5.41DS.$$

A_s represents the accommodative effort required to overcome this divergence of light from the artificial near point position.

$$A_s = -\bar{L}_{lens} \left(\bar{L}_1 \text{ in the diagram}\right)$$
$$\bar{L}_1 = -4D$$
$$\therefore A_s = -(-4) = 4DS$$

∴ Spectacle accommodation = +4DS

Ocular accommodation, $A_{oc,max} = K - B$ (B is L_2 in the diagram)

$$L_1 = L_1 + F = -4 + (-5.41) = -9.41D$$
$$L_2 = \frac{L_1}{(1 - dL_1)}$$
$$L_2 = \frac{-9.41}{1 - (0.015 \times -9.41)} = -8.25D$$

$$\therefore A_{oc} = -5 - (-8.25)$$

∴ Ocular accommodation = +3.25D

[ii] Retinal image size, $h' = h \times \dfrac{\bar{L}_1}{\bar{L}_1{'}} \times \dfrac{\bar{L}_2}{\bar{L}_2{'}}$

$$\therefore h' = 17.11 \times \frac{-4}{-9.41} \times \frac{-8.25}{+60} = -1.000mm$$

∴ Retinal image size = –1mm.

[b] [i] <u>Spectacle accommodation = +4.00D (as in [a])</u>

$$F_v' = \frac{+5}{1 + (0.015 \times 5)} = +4.65DS$$

Hypermetropia is refractive, $\therefore \overline{K}' = +60D$

$A_{oc} = K - B = 5.00 - B$

$\overline{L}_1 = -4.00D; \quad L_1' = -4.00 + 4.65 = +0.65D$

$\overline{L}_2 = \dfrac{0.65}{1 - (0.015 \times 0.65)} = +0.66D$

$\therefore A_{oc} = +5.00 - 0.66 = +4.34D$

$\therefore$ <u>Ocular accommodation = +4.34D</u>

[ii] Retinal image size = $17.11 \times \dfrac{-4.00}{+0.65} \times \dfrac{0.66}{60} = \underline{-1.158mm}$

42. A subject with a PD of 60*mm* is corrected by R. & L. –8.75DS @ 13*mm*.

    [a] Determine the ocular refraction

    [b] If the ocular amplitude of accommodation is 8D, find the positions of the true near and far points of accommodation.

    [c] The subject now views, corrected, an object on the midline, 40*cm* from the spectacle plane. If the centres of rotation are 25*mm* behind the spectacle plane, calculate the convergence required to view this object. Specify your answer in [i] degrees [ii] prism dioptres [iii] metre angles.

[a]

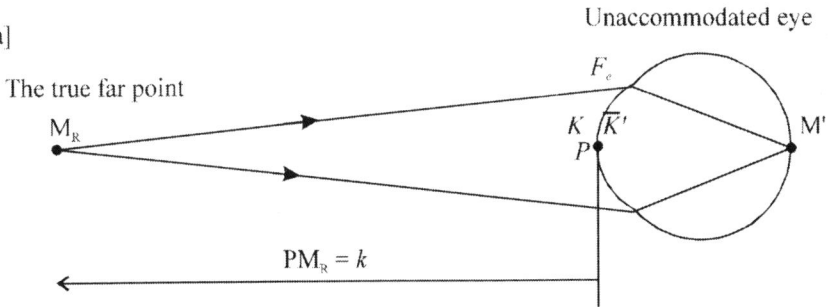

[b]

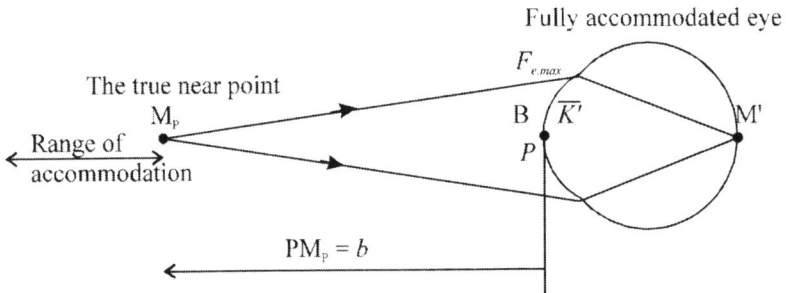

[a] $F_v' = F = -8.75DS$ $d = 13mm$

$$K = \frac{F}{(1-dF)} = \frac{-8.75}{1-(0.013\times-8.75)} = -7.86D$$

∴ Ocular refraction = −7.86D

[b] $A_{oc} = 8.00D$ $A_{oc} = K - B$

∴ $B = K - A_{oc} = -7.86 - 8.00 = -15.86D$

∴ $b = -6.305cm$ [true near point]

True far point $= \dfrac{1}{K} = \dfrac{1}{-7.86} = -12.723cm$

∴ Positions of true near and far points are at −6.305cm and −12.723cm respectively.

[c] [i]

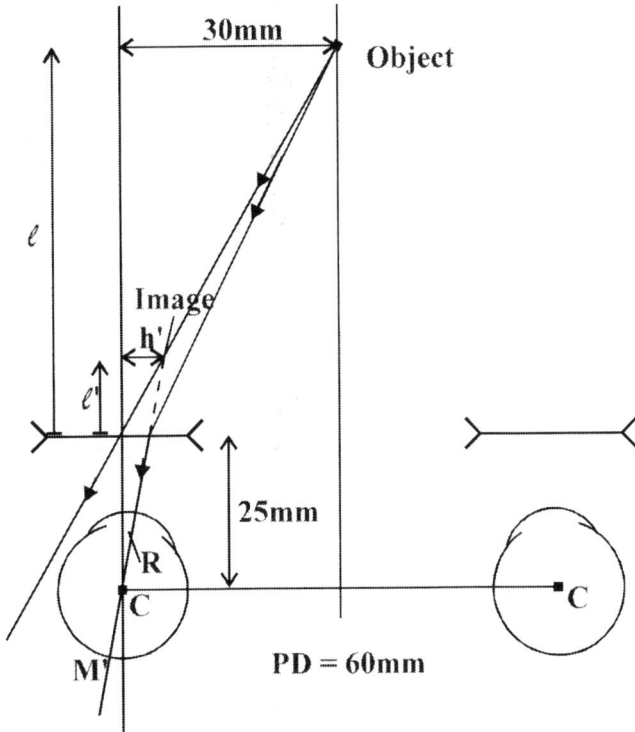

To find image distance l′:

$\ell = -40cm \qquad \therefore L = -2.5D \quad F \qquad = \qquad -8.75DS$

$\therefore L' = -2.5 - 8.75 = -11.25D$

$\ell' = \dfrac{100}{-11.25} = -8.89cm$

From the diagram: $\tan R = \dfrac{h'}{(-\ell'+25)}$

Find h' by similar Δs, where $\dfrac{h'}{30} = \dfrac{\ell'}{\ell}$

$$\therefore h' = \frac{30 \times -88.9}{-400} = 6.67mm$$

$$\therefore \tan R = \frac{6.67}{-(88.9+25)} = \frac{6.67}{-113.9}$$

$$\therefore R = 3.35°$$

$\therefore$ <u>Convergence required for each eye = 3.35°</u>

[ii] To find convergence in prism dioptres: $P = 100.\tan R$
$$= 5.86\Delta$$

$\therefore$ <u>Convergence required for each eye = 5.86Δ</u>

[iii] Convergence in MA $= \dfrac{1}{d} = \dfrac{1000}{(400+25)} = 2.35MA$

---

43. An eye with 5D of refractive myopia has a near point at 6.5cm.
[a] What is the amplitude of accommodation and range of clear vision?
[b] Find the retinal image size for an object 5mm high.

---

[a]

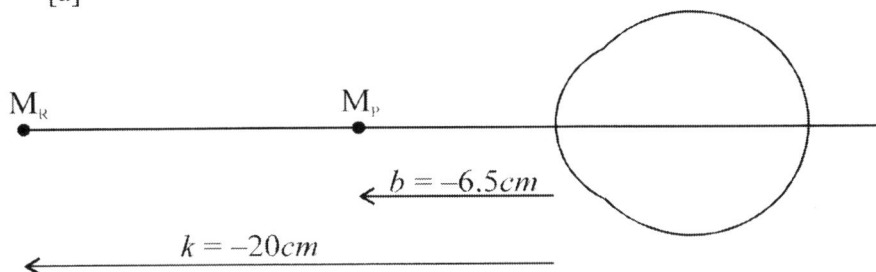

$A_{oc} = K - B$ where $K = -5D$ and $b = -6.5cm$.

$\therefore B = -15.38D$

$\therefore A_{oc} = -5 - (-15.38) = +10.38D$

$\therefore$ Amplitude of accommodation is $10.38D$

The far point is at $-20cm$ since $K = -5D$

$\therefore$ Range of clear vision extends from $-20cm$ to $-6.5cm$.

[b] To find retinal image size, h', use $h' = \dfrac{h \times L_{eye}}{\overline{K}'}$ where $L_{eye} = B$

and $\overline{K}' = +60D$ since eye is refractively ametropic

$\therefore h' = 5 \times \dfrac{-15.38}{+60} = -1.28mm$

---

44. A subject viewing an object at $1/3m$ has a pupil diameter of 4mm. If a blur disc size of 0.028mm is not noticeable, calculate the dioptric and linear depth of field. Assume a standard reduced eye which has accommodated by 3.00D.

Blur disc diameter $y = 0.028mm$ Pupil size $p = 4mm$

Standard Reduced eye has accommodated by 3.00D so the power is now $+63.00D$

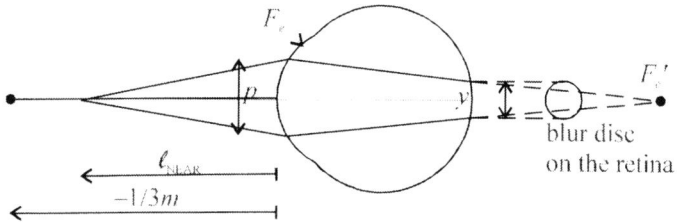

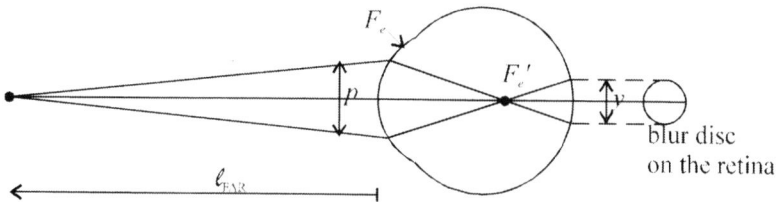

Object at $1/3m$, ℓ_{NEAR} is the nearer position which produces a blur circle size of y and ℓ_{FAR} is the further position.

Using the blur circle formula for a near object

$$y = \frac{p[K'-L']}{K'} \text{ gives } 0.028 = \frac{4[60-L']}{60}$$

$$0.42 = [60 - L']$$

Now $L' = L + F_e$ So $0.42 = [60 - (L + 63)]$

which gives $L = -3 \pm 0.42D$

The dioptric depth of field is therefore $\pm 0.42D$

The nearest position for the object has the vergence
$L_{NEAR} = -3.00 - 0.42D = -3.42D$ so the distance
ℓ_{NEAR} is $100/-3.42 = -29.24cm$

The furthest position has the vergence
$L_{FAR} = -3.00 + 0.42 = -2.58D$ so the distance
ℓ_{FAR} is $100/-2.58 = -38.76cm$

So the linear depth of field is from $-38.76cm$ to $-29.24cm$
$= 9.52cm$

45. Find the positions of the true and artificial far and near points for an eye with an ocular refraction of $-8.00D$ and an amplitude of accommodation of $3.00D$. The eye is corrected for distance vision by a lens placed $12mm$ from the reduced surface.

$K = -8.00D$ So $k = 100/-8 = -12.5cm$ (True far point)

$Amp = +3.00D$
$Amp = K - B$ So $B = K - Amp = -8 - 3 = -11.00D$
$b = 100/-11 = -9.09cm$ (True near point)

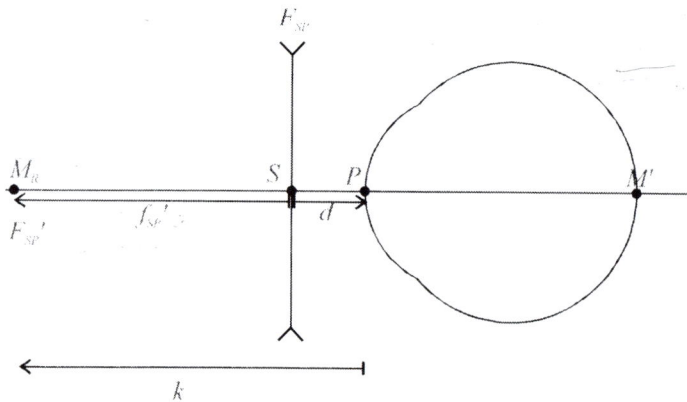

$d = 12mm = 1.2cm$

$f_{SP}' =$
$-11.3cm$
So F_{SP}'
$= -8.85D$

When the eye is corrected for distance vision and is unaccommodated, the point conjugate with the macula is infinity so this is location of the artificial far point. The lens will form an image of an object at infinity at the eye's true far point.

To find the artificial near point it is necessary to find the object position to produce an image at the eye's true near point. This means stepping backwards from the eye through the lens.

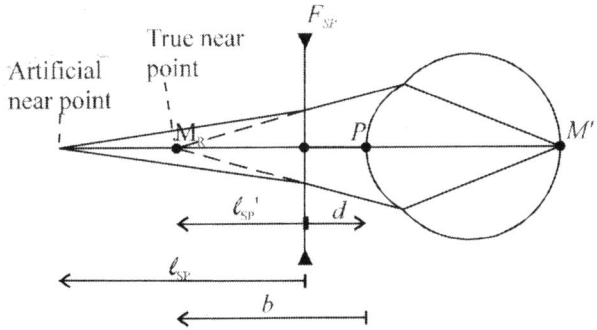

$b = -9.09cm$

$d = 1.2cm$

$\ell_{SP}' = -7.89cm$

So

$L_{SP}' = 100/-7.89$

$= -12.67D$

$F_{SP} = -8.85D$

$L_{SP} = L_{SP}' - F_{SP} = -12.67 - (-8.85) = -3.82D$

$\ell_{SP} = 100/-3.82 = -26.18cm$ (Artificial near point)

46. Estimate the addition that might be required by a patient with 2.00D of accommodation who has near working distance of 1/3m. Explain the basis on which this estimate is made. If the subject is emmetropic find the position of the far and near points and the range of clear vision. If the estimated addition is worn in the form of a contact lens (this means the vertex distance can be assumed to be zero) find the position of the artificial far and near points and the range of clear vision.

Near working distance of 1/3m requires 3.00D of accommodation.

The subject has an amplitude of 2.00D. It would not be comfortable for the subject to use all of the available accommodation, so it is usual to require only 2/3 of the amplitude to be used. So the subject can supply 2/3 of 2.00D = 1.33D. The remaining 1.67D that is necessary for clear vision at 1/3m must be given in the form of an Addition.

Thus the estimated Addition is +1.75D.

Emmetropic subject So $K = 0$ and $k = \infty$ (True far point)

Amp = 2.00 So $B = K - Amp = 0 - 2.00 = -2.00D$
$b = 100/-2.00 = -50cm$ (True near point)

Range of clear vision is from ∞ to $-50cm$.

When wearing the
Addition of +1.75D
the
unaccommodated
eye is effectively
myopic by 1.75D
and is therefore
focused at
−57.14cm (Artificial far point)

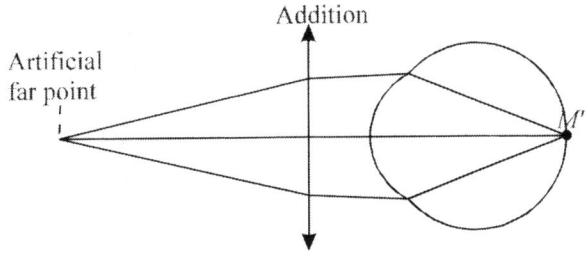

Artificial
far point

Addition

M'

When fully
accommodated the
eye is effectively
myopic by 3.75D
(1.75 + 2.00) and is
therefore focused at
100/−3.75 = −26.67cm
(Artificial near point)
Range of clear vision through Addition is from
−57.14cm to −26.67cm
= 30.47cm.

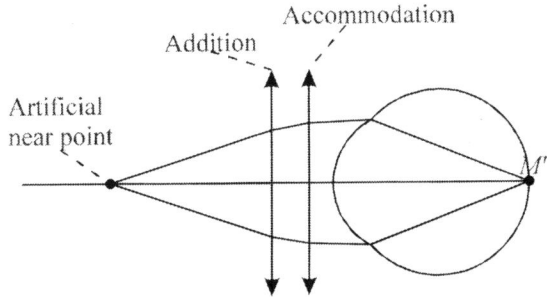

Accommodation

Addition

Artificial
near point

M'

47. An eye with the ocular refraction of Plano/+4.00 × 90 views a distant object in the form of a thin wire cross. Describe and explain the form of the retinal image if the eye is
[a] unaccommodated   [b] accommodates by 2.00D
[c] accommodates by 4.00D [d] accommodates by 4.50D.

$K = 0.00/+4.00 \times 90 = 0.00 \times 180/+4.00 \times 90$

[a] As $K \times 180 = 0.00$ the horizontal focal line is on the retina when the eye is unaccommodated. The vertical line is behind the retina   The retinal image is made up of horizontal lines so the vertical bar of the cross is blurred.

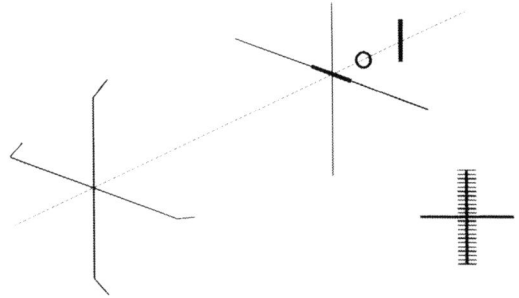

[b] When eye accommodates it increases its power and moves the focal lines forwards. 2.00D of accommodation brings the circle of least confusion onto the retina, so both bars of the cross are equally blurred.

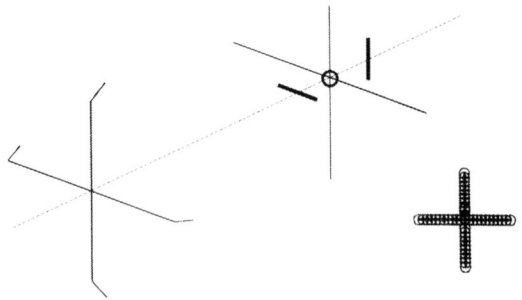

[c] 4.00*D* of
accommodation moves
the vertical focal line
onto the retina. The
retinal image is made up
of vertical lines and the
horizontal bar of the
cross is blurred.

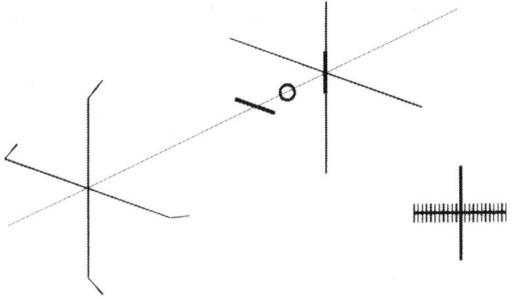

[d] 4.50*D* of
accommodation moves
the vertical line in front
of the retina. The
retinal image of each
point on the cross is in
the form of a vertical
ellipse, so both bars are
blurred but the vertical bar is less blurred than the horizontal.

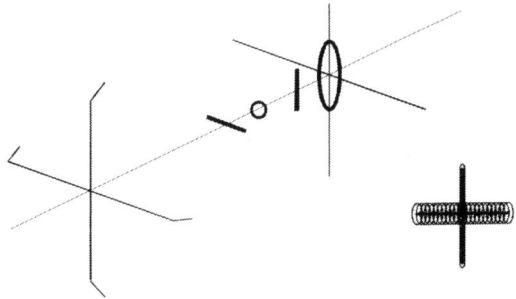

48. An eye has a reduced surface power of +61.00D and an axial length of +23.50mm. Calculate the power of the lens placed at 15mm required to correct this eye for distance vision and the spectacle magnification produced.
Find the size of the retinal image if the corrected eye views a 36m Snellen letter at a distance of 6m.

$k' = +23.50mm$ $\bar{K}' = n'/k'$
$= (4/3 \times 1000)/23.50$
$= +56.74D$

$F_e = +61.00D$ $K = \bar{K}' - F_e$
$= 56.74 - 61.00$
$= -4.26D$

$k = 1/K$
$= 100/-4.26$
$= -23.47cm$

$d = 15mm$
$= 1.5cm$

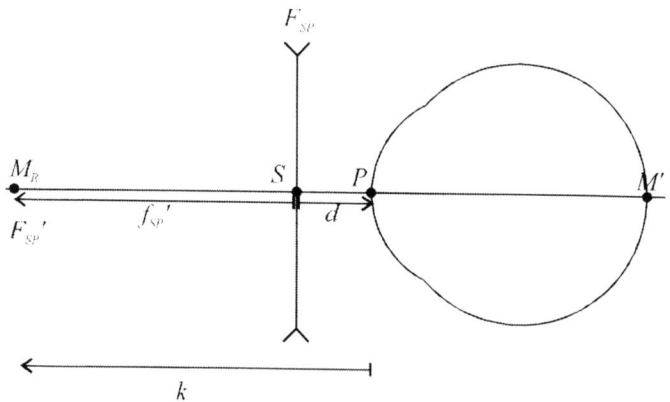

From diagram

$f_{SP}' = -21.97cm$

$F_{SP} = 1/f_{SP}' = 100/-21.97$
$= -4.55D$

$SM = K/F_{SP} = -4.26/-4.55 = 0.936$

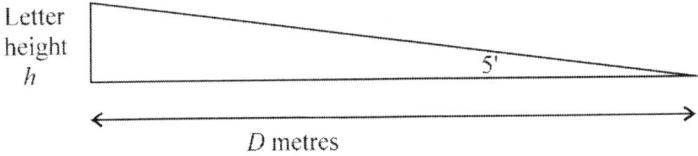

From diagram

$h = 36000 \times \tan 5'$
$\quad = 52.36 mm$

$\tan \omega_0 = 52.36/6000$

$h_u{}'$
$= -(1000 \times \tan \omega_0)/K'$
$= -\left(1000 \times \dfrac{52.36}{6000}\right) \div 56.74$
$= -0.154 mm$

$h_c{}' = h_u{}' \times SM$
$\quad = -0.154 \times 0.936$
$\quad = -0.144 mm$

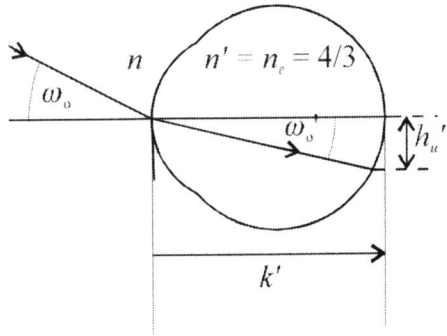

49. If an eye is corrected for distance by +10.00D at 12*mm*, how much ocular accommodation is required to view an object at 33.33*cm* from the lens?
What is the nearest point that can be seen clearly by the corrected eye if the amplitude of accommodation is 5.00D?

Estimating ocular accommodation required

For a distance of 33.33*cm*, accommodation will be approximately +3.00D. As the subject is a corrected hypermetrope it is to be expected that the calculated value will be greater than +3.00D.

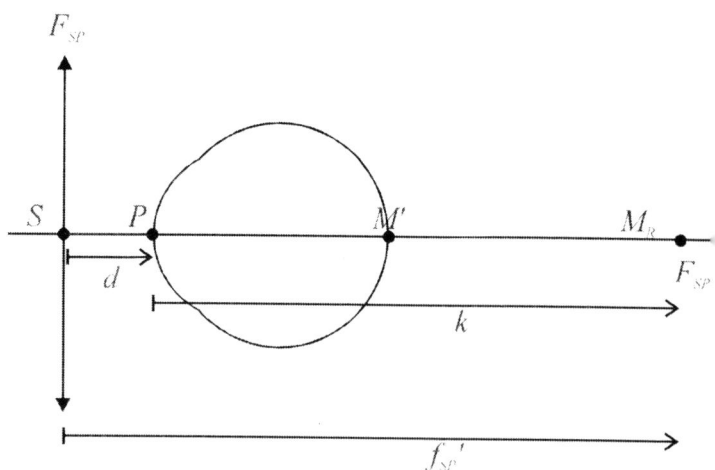

To find K

$F_{SP} = +10.00D$ $f_{SP}' = 100/10 = +10cm$

$d = 12mm = 1.2cm$

From diagram
$k = +8.8cm$

$K = 100/8.8 = +11.36D$

To find L_e
$\ell_{SP} = -33.33cm$
$L_{SP} = 100/-33.33 = -3.00D$

$L_{SP}' = L_{SP} + F_{SP} = -3.00 + 10.00 = +7.00D$

$\ell_{SP}' = 100/7$
$= +14.29cm$

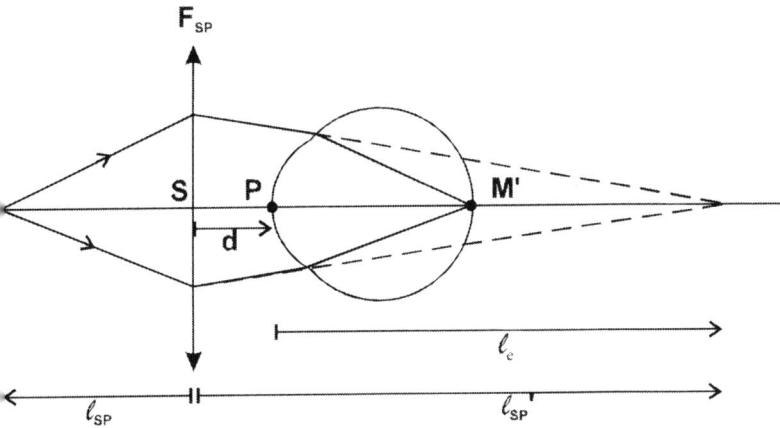

From diagram
$\ell_e = +13.09cm$
$L_e = 100/13.09 = +7.64D$

To find A

$A = K - L_e = 11.36 - 7.64$
$$= +3.72D$$

This calculation is the reverse of the first part. The accommodation used is given, it is required to find the object distance.

For an eye using $5.00D$ of accommodation the working distance would be approximately $-20cm$. The effect of the accommodation is reduced by the positive lens, so the calculated value will be numerically greater than $-20cm$.

Amp. $= +5.00D$
Using $A = K - L_e$ (or $Amp = K - B$)
$L_e = K - A = 11.36 - 5$
$$= +6.36D$$
$\ell_e = 100/6.36 = +15.72cm$

From diagram
$\ell_{SP}' = +16.92cm$
$L_{SP}' = 100/16.92 = +5.91D$

$F_{SP} = +10.00D$
$L_{SP} = L_{SP}' - F_{SP} = 5.91 - 10$
$$= -4.09D$$

$\ell_{SP} = 100/-4.09 = -24.45cm$
So the object distance is $-24.45cm$

---

50. Calculate the ocular refraction for a reduced eye which has an axial length of +20.50*mm* and radii of curvature of +5.71*mm* along 60 and +5.39*mm* along 150.. What type of astigmatism does this eye have ?
Calculate the powers of the spectacle lens required to correct this eye when placed at
a) 10*mm* and b) 16*mm*.

$k' = +20.50mm$

$$\overline{K'} = \frac{n'}{k'} = \frac{4/3}{0.0205} = +65.04D$$

The direction of the radii of curvature gives the power meridians, so the axes are at 90° to these.

Axis 60
$r = +5.39mm$
$F_e = (n' - n)/r$
$$F_e = \frac{(4/3 - 1)}{0.00539}$$
$= +61.84D$

Axis 150
$r = +5.71mm$
$$F_e = \frac{(4/3 - 1)}{0.00571}$$
$= +58.38D$

$K = \overline{K'} - F_e$
$= 65.04 - 61.84$
$= +3.20D$

$K = 65.04 - 58.38$
$= +6.66D$

Ocular refraction is $+3.20D \times 60/+6.66D \times 150$
$= +3.20/+3.46 \times 150$
The eye has compound hypermetropic astigmatism, against-the-rule.

To find F_{SP} at 9mm

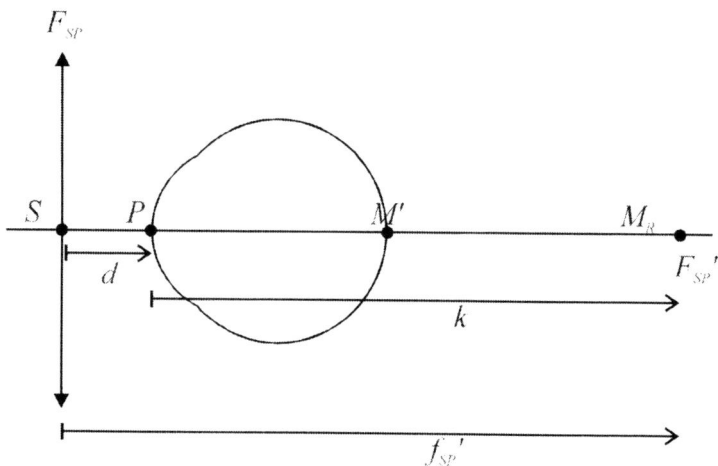

$k = l/K = 100/3.20$
   $= +31.25cm$

$k = 100/6.66$
   $= +15.02cm$

$d = 10mm = 1cm$

$f_{SP}' = +32.25cm$

$f_{SP}' = +16.02cm$

$F_{SP} = 1/f_{SP}' = 100/32.25$
   $= +3.10D$

$F_{SP} = 100/16.02$
   $= +6.24D$

So F_{SP} at 10mm is $+3.10 \times 60/+6.24 \times 150 = +3.10/+3.14 \times 150$

To find F_{SP} at 16mm

$d = 16mm = 1.6cm$

$f_{SP}' = +32.85cm$ $f_{SP}' = +16.62cm$

$F_{SP} = 100/32.85$ $F_{SP} = 100/16.62$
      $= +3.04D$ $= +6.02D$

So Fsp at $16mm$ is $+3.04D \times 60/+6.02D \times 150 = +3.04/+2.98 \times$ 150

Note that the sphere and the cylinder change by different amounts when the back vertex distance is altered.

51. A standard reduced emmetropic eye views an object placed 25cm from a +2.50D lens which is 12mm from the reduced surface. How much ocular accommodation is required ? If the object is 5mm high, find the retinal image size.

Emmetropic subject wearing +2.50DS (reading spectacles) viewing an object at 25cm. If no lens was being used, the accommodation required would be approximately 4.00D but this requirement will be reduced by the +2.50D lens to around 1.50D.

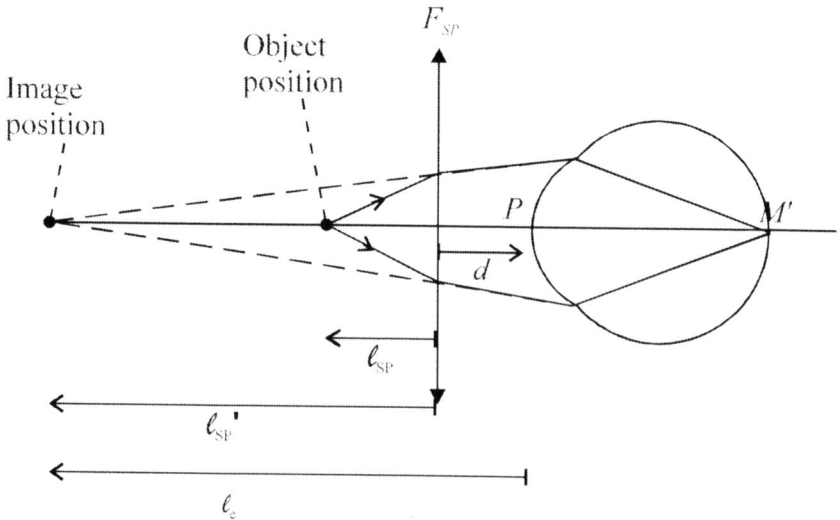

The eye has to accommodate to focus on the image formed by the lens, so the position of this image must first be found.

$\ell_{SP} = -25cm \; L_{SP} = -4.00D$

$L_{SP}' = L_{SP} + F_{SP} = -4 + 2.5 = -1.50D$

$\ell_{SP}' = 1/L_{SP}' = 100/-1.5 = -66.67cm$

$d = 12mm = 1.2cm$

so using diagram

$\ell_e = -67.87cm$

$L_e = 100/-67.87 = -1.47D$

$A = K - L_e = 0 - (-1.47) = +1.47D$

So accommodation required is $1.47D$

To find the retinal image size

$h'' = h \times m_l \times m_2$ where m_1 is the magnification of the lens and m_2 is the magnification due to the eye.

So $h'' = h \times L_{SP}/L_{SP}' \times L_e/L_e' = h \times L_{SP}/L_{SP}' \times L_e/\overline{K}'$
$h = 5mm$

$h'' = 5 \times -4/-1.5 \times -1.47/60$
$\quad = -0.327mm$

52. A subject can just resolve grating bars of width 1*mm* at a distance of 1.1459*m*. Calculate the Minimum Angle of Resolution. What would be the Snellen acuity for a chart at 6*m* ?

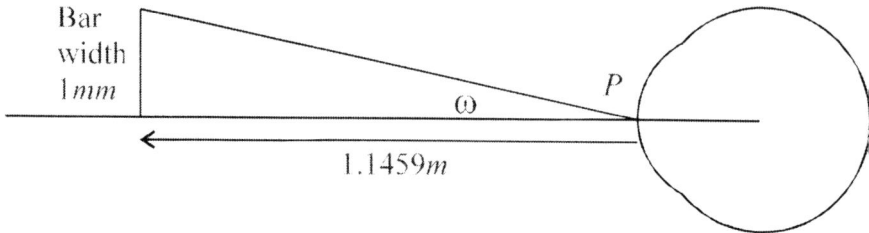

Minimum Angle of Resolution (ω) is the angle subtended by one bar of the grating at the eye.

So tan ω = 1/1145.9
ω = 3 minutes

Find Snellen acuity by MAR

VA = $1/\omega$ = 1/3

Snellen acuity = 1/3 × 6/6 = 6/18

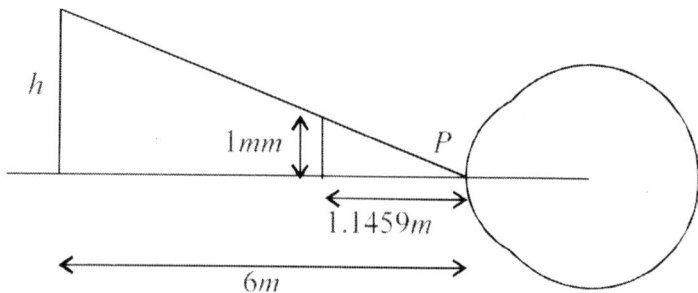

OR Using similar triangles

Bar width resolved at 6m

$$= \frac{1}{1.1459} \times 6 = 5.236mm$$

Letter height is 5×5.236
$= 26.18mm$

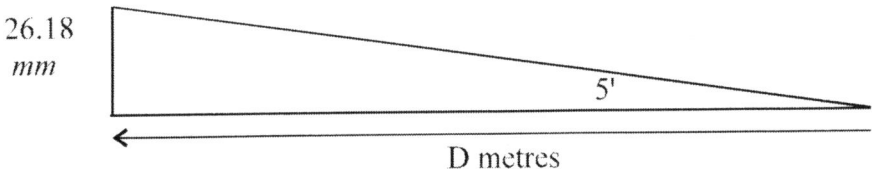

This letter subtends 5' at 26.18/tan 5'
$$= 18000mm$$
$$= 18m$$

Snellen acuity $= 6/18$

> **53.** An axially ametropic eye views a 1*cm* high object at a distance
> of 6*m*. If the ocular ametropia is –3.00*D* and the pupil
> diameter is 2*mm* calculate
>   a) the axial length
>   b) the blur circle size
>   c) the total retinal image size
> If this eye is corrected by a lens at 13*mm*, calculate
>   d) the power of the lens
>   e) the spectacle magnification produced
>   f) the retinal image size in the corrected eye

a) Axial ametropia so $F_c = +60.00D$

$$K = -3.00D \quad K' = \overline{K}' + F_c = -3.00 + 60$$
$$= +57.00D$$

$$k' = n'/\overline{K}' = (1000 \times 4/3)/57 = +23.392mm$$

Formation of blur circle

b) $\ell = -6m$

$L = 1/\ell$

$= -0.17D$

$L' = L + F_c$

$= -0.17 + 60$

$= +59.83D$

$p = 2mm$

$$y = p\left[\frac{K'-L'}{K'}\right]$$

$$= 2\left[\frac{57 - 59.83}{57}\right]$$

$$= -0.099mm$$

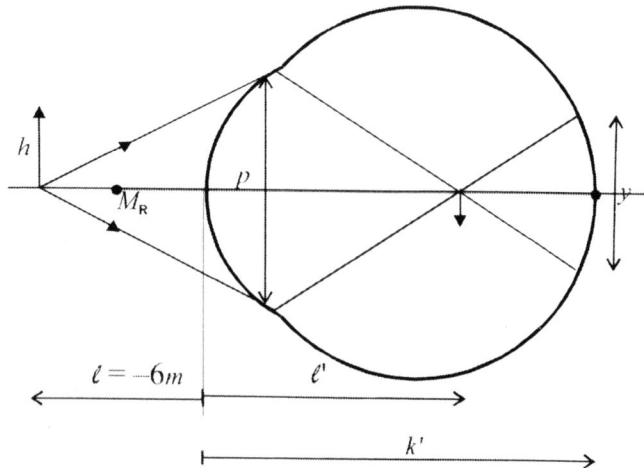

$\ell = -6m$ ℓ'

k'

c) Total retinal image size $= y + h_u{}'$

Uncorrected retinal image $h_u{}'$

$h_u{}' = -(\tan \omega)/K'$
$\tan \omega = h/\ell = 1/600$
$h_u{}' = -(1/600)/57$
$= -0.000029m$
$= -0.029mm.$

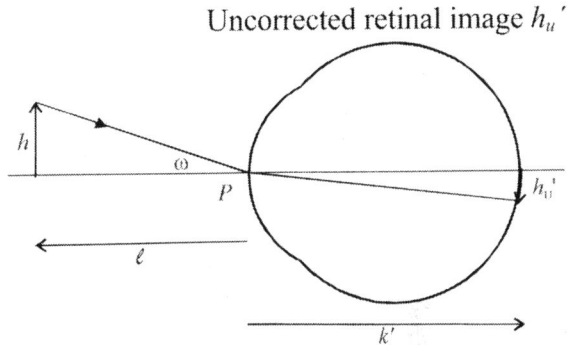

TRIS
$= 0.099 + 0.029$
$= 0.128mm$

d) $K = -3.00D \quad k = \dfrac{100}{-3} = -33.33cm$

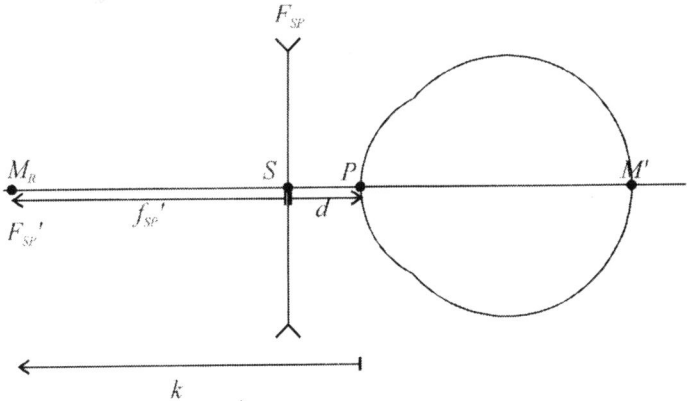

$d = 15mm = 1.5cm$

$f_{SP}{}' = -31.83cm$

$F_{SP} = 100/-31.83$
$= -3.14D$

e) $SM = K/F_{SP}$
$= -3.0/-3.14 = 0.955$

f) $h_c{}' = h_u{}' \times SM$
$= -0.029 \times 0.955$
$= -0.028mm$

93

> **54.** A simple optometer has a test target 2*mm* high and a thin +10.00*D* lens. If the optometer lens is 12*mm* from the reduced surface, find the target position and retinal image size when the instrument is correctly focused for
>   a) an axial hyperope who would be corrected for distance by +6.00 at 16*mm*
>   b) an axial myope who would be corrected for distance vision by –6.00D at 16*mm*.

When the target is in the correct position, the image of it formed by the optometer lens must be at the eye's far point to produce a clear retinal image.

$\ell' = f_{SP}'$ and so $L' = F_{SP}$.

L (and therefore ℓ) can be found from $L' = L + F_{OPT}$.

The retinal image size can be found by magnification

e.g. $h'' = h \times m_1 \times m_2$ where m_1 is the magnification of the optometer lens and m_2 is the magnification of the eye.

So $h'' = h \times m_{OPT} \times m_e = h \times L/L' \times L_e/L_e'$

The image formed by the optometer lens is at the eye's far point and this acts as the object for the eye so $\ell_e = k$ and $L_e = K$. The final image is on the retina giving $\ell_e' = k'$ and $L_e' = \overline{K}'$,

Thus $h'' = h \times L/L' \times K/\overline{K}'$

a) To find the target position

    $F_{SP} = +6.00D = L'$

    $L = L' - F_{OPT} = 6 - 10 = -4.00D$
    $\ell = 100/-4 = -25cm$

Target position is $-25cm$.

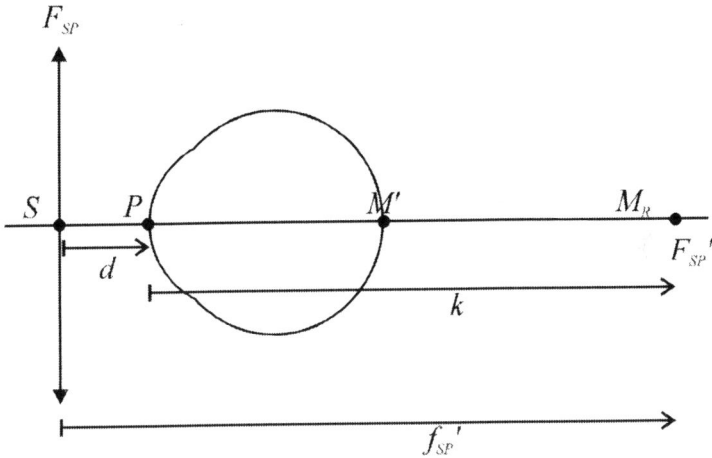

To find the retinal image size

$f_{SP}' = 100/6 = +16.67cm$
$d = 12mm = 1.2cm$

Using diagram to find K
$k = +15.47cm$

$K = 100/15.47 = +6.46D$

Axial ametropia so $F_e = +60.00D$
$K' = K + F_e = +66.46D$

$h'' = h \times L/L' \times K/K'$
$$= 2 \times \frac{-4}{6} \times \frac{6.46}{66.46}$$
$$= -0.130mm$$

b) To find the target position

$$F_{SP} = -6.00D = L'$$

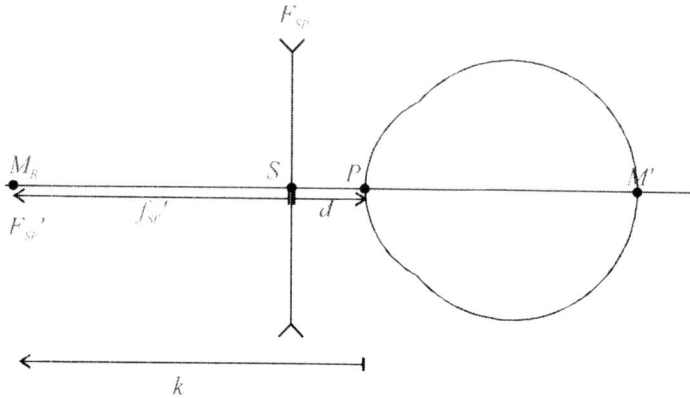

$$L = -6 - 10 = -16.00D$$
$$\ell = 100/-16 = -6.25cm$$

The target position is $-6.25cm$

To find the retinal image size
$$f_{SP}' = -16.67cm$$
$$d = 1.2cm$$

From diagram $k = -17.87cm$

$$K = 100/-17.87 = -5.60D$$

$$K' = 60 + (-5.60) = 54.40D$$

$$h'' = 2 \times -16/-6 \times -5.60/54.40$$

$$= -0.549mm$$

55. A thin +12.00D lens is used as a Badal optometer to measure spectacle refraction. What is the subject's spectacle refraction if the target is placed +5cm from the first principal focus of the optometer lens?

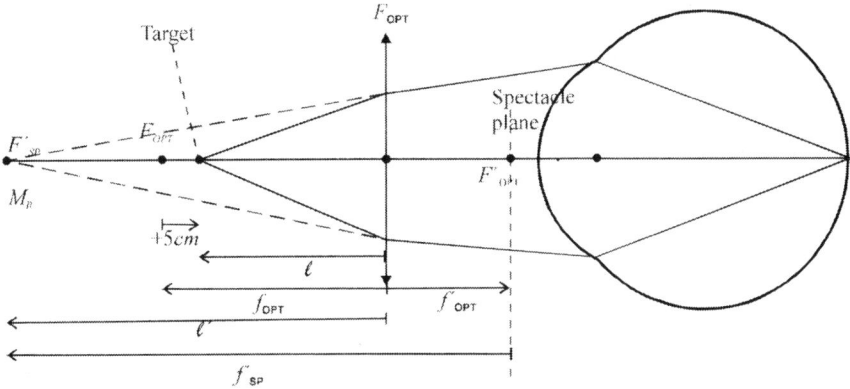

$F_{OPT} = +12.00D$ $f_{OPT} = -n/F_{OPT} = -100/12 = -8.33cm$

Target is +5cm from first principal focus so $\ell = -3.33cm$

$L = 100/-3.33 = -30.00D$

$L' = L + F_{OPT} = -30.00 + 12.00 = -18.00D$

$\ell' = 100/-18.00 = -5.56cm$

The spectacle point is at the second principal focus of the optometer lens, that is at +8.33cm. The distance from the spectacle point S to the image formed by the optometer lens is the focal length f'_{SP} of the distance correcting lens F_{SP}.

From diagram

$F'_{SP} = -13.89cm$, so $F_{SP} = 100/-13.89 = -7.20D$.

Alternatively using Newton's relation

$$F_{SP} = -x\, F^2_{OPT}$$

$F_{OPT} = +12.00D$ and $x = +5cm$

So $F_{SP} = -0.05 \times 12^2 = -7.20D$

56. A reduced eye has an ocular ametropia of +5.00D and an amplitude of accommodation of 6.00D. It is corrected for distance vision by a thin lens placed at 15mm. Find the power of this lens and the positions of the apparent far and near points.
Find the position of the apparent far and near points when this eye looks through a thin +8.00DS lens 15mm from the eye.

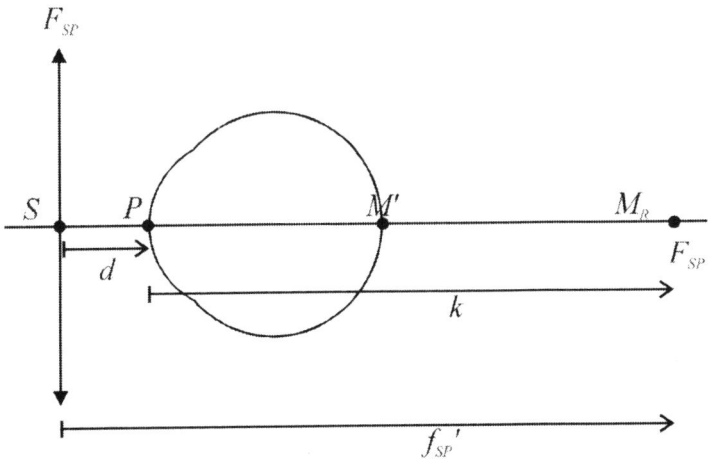

$K = +5.00D$ $k = 100/5 = +20cm$

$d = 15mm = 1.5cm$

From diagram
$f_{SP}' = +21.5cm$
$F_{SP} = 100/21.5 = +4.65D$

Apparent far point is at ∞ when the eye is wearing its distance correcting lens.

Estimating the position of the apparent near point, the amplitude is +6.00D so the position will be approximately $100/-6 = -16.7cm$. As the eye is hyperopic it is expected that the positive lens will reduce the effect of the accommodation so the actual distance will be greater than the estimated value.

To find apparent near point accurately it is necessary to ray–trace back from the real near point to find the object position.

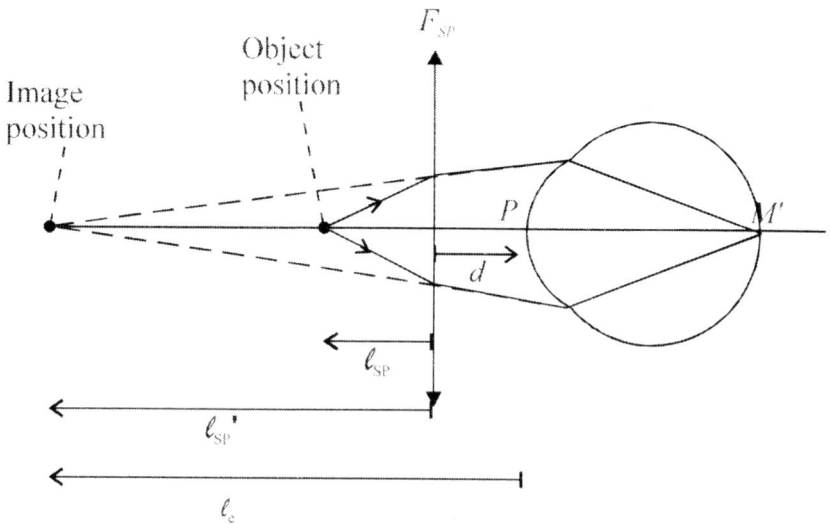

The apparent near point is the object position

To find the real near point

Using $A = K - L_e$ (or $Amp = K - B$)

$L_e = K - A = 5 - 6 = -1.00D$

$\ell_e = 100/-1 = -1m$ (this is the real near point distance)
$d = 15mm = 1.5cm$

From diagram $\ell_{SP}' = -98.5cm$

$L_{SP}' = 100/-98.5 = -1.02D$

$L_{SP} = L_{SP}' - F_{SP} = -1.02 - 4.65$
$\quad = -5.67D$

So the apparent near point is at $100/-5.67 = -17.64cm$

With the $+8.00D$ lens

This is $3.35D$ stronger than the distance correction, so both the apparent far and near points will be $3.00D$ closer. Thus the apparent far point will be at approximately $-1/3m$ and the apparent near point will be at approximately $-9.00D$ which is $-11.11cm$.

The exact position of the apparent far point is found by ray tracing back from the real far point.

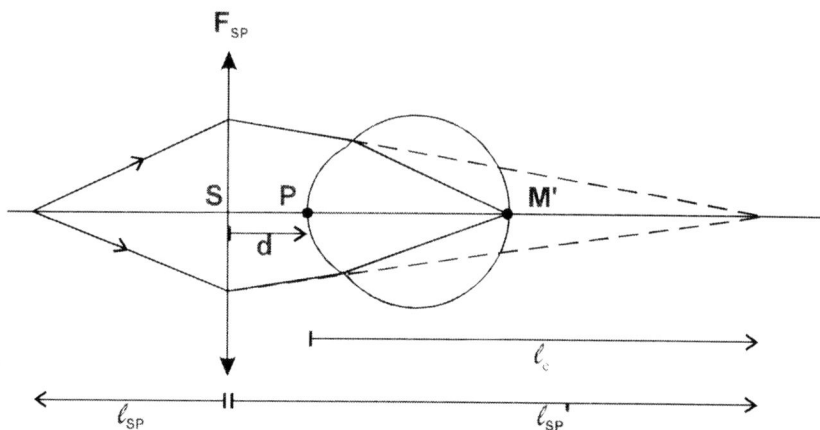

$k = +20cm$ and $d = 1.5cm$

Using diagram

$\ell_{SP}' = +21.5cm$

$L_{SP}' = +4.65D$

So $L_{SP} = +4.65 - 8 = -3.35D$

$\ell_{SP} = 100/-3.35 = -29.85cm$

The apparent far point position is $-29.85cm$

To find the apparent near point

As in diagram $\ell_{SP}' = -98.5cm$ So $L_{SP}' = -1.02D$

$L_{SP} = -1.02 - 8 = -9.02D$
So the apparent near point is at $\ell_{SP} = 100/-9.02 = -11.09cm$

57. If the refractive index of a reduced eye is 1.305 and it has an axial length of +23.85*mm* and the radius of curvature of the reduced surface is +4.824*mm* calculate the power of the surface and the ocular ametropia.

Find the power of the lens and its distance from the reduced surface if the eye is corrected for distance by a lens which produces a spectacle magnification of 0.895..

The corrected eye views a distant object which subtends an angle of 3Δ Calculate the retinal image size.

$r = + 4.824mm$ and $n' = 1.305$
$F_e = (n' - n)/r = 1000(1.305 - 1)/4.824 = +63.23D$

$k' = +23.85mm$

$K' = n'/k' = (1000 \times 1.305)/23.85 = +54.72D$

$K = \overline{K'} - F_e = 54.72 - 63.23 = -8.51D$

$SM = 0.895$

$SM = K/F_{SP}$ So $F_{SP} = K/SM = -8.51/0.895 = -9.51D$

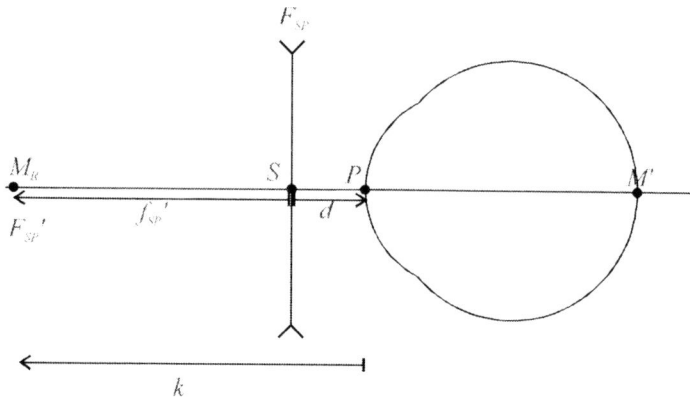

$K = -8.51D$ $k = 100/-8.5 = -11.75cm$

$F_{SP} = -9.51$ $f_{SP}' = 100/-9.51 = -10.52cm$

So $d = -10.52 - (-11.75) = 1.23cm$

$\omega = 3\Delta$ So $\tan \omega_b = 3/100$

To find the corrected retinal image size

$h_c' = h_u' \times SM$

$h_u' = -1000(\tan \omega)/\overline{K}' = -1000 \times (3/100)/54.72$
    $= -0.548mm$

$h_c' = -0.548 \times 0.895 = -0.491mm$

58. A reduced eye has an ocular ametropia of $+5.00/-3.00 \times 90$ and an axial length of $+19.60mm$. Find the power of the reduced surface if $n_e = 4/3$.

The eye has a pupil diameter of $4mm$ and views a distant point object. Calculate the dimensions of the blur ellipse on the retina and draw a sketch to indicate its orientation.

$K = +5.00/-3.00 \times 90 = +5.00 \times 180/+2.00 \times 90$

$k' = +19.60mm$

$\overline{K}' = n'/k' = (4/3 \times 1000)/19.6 = +68.03D$

Axis 180

$K = +5.00D$
$K' = +68.03D$
$F_e = \overline{K}' - K$
$\quad = 68.03 - 5.00$
$\quad = +63.03D$

Axis 90

$K = +2.00D$
$\overline{K}' = +68.03D$

$F_e = 68.03 - 2.00$
$\quad = 66.03D$

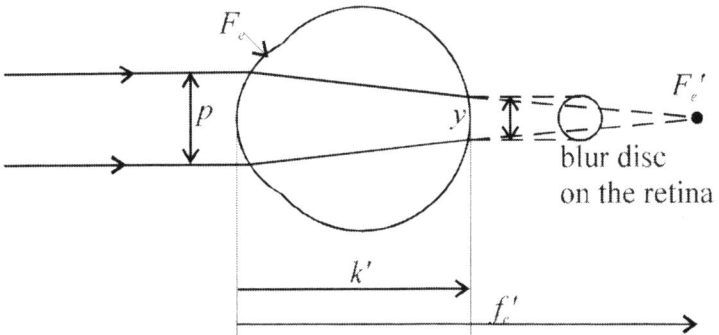

blur disc on the retina

So $F_c = +63.03/+3.00 \times 90$

As it is a distant object the formula $y = pK/\overline{K}'$ can be used to find the blur dimensions.

$p = 4mm$

$y = 4 \times 5/68.03$ $y = 4 \times 2/68.03$
    $= 0.294mm$ $= 0.118mm$

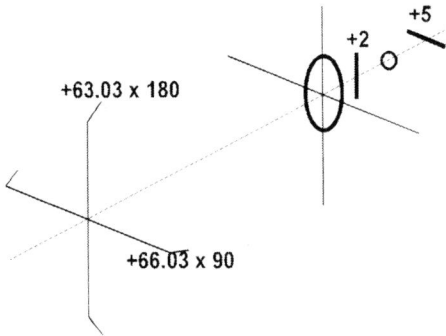

+63.03 x 180

+66.03 x 90

+2

+5

From diagram the vertical focal line will be nearer the retina so the long axis of the blur ellipse is along $90°$.

0.118mm wide

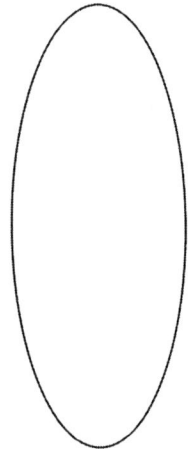

0.294mm high

---

59. A +6.00D lens is at a distance of 14mm from the reduced surface of an unaccommodated axially ametropic eye. An object is placed 12.5cm in front of the lens. If the image on the retina is sharp, calculate the ocular refraction and the axial length of the eye.

The +6.00D lens is now placed 14mm from the reduced surface of an unaccommodated eye with ocular refraction of +1.95D. Where must the object be placed to produce a clear retinal image?

The object that is seen clearly is not at infinity so the lens is not the distance correcting lens. Although not stated, this problem can be regarded as a simple optometer question. The image formed by the lens will be at the eye's far point, so it is necessary to find this position.

$\ell = -12.5cm$ $L = 100/-12.5 = -8.00D$

$F = +6.00D$ So $L' = -8.00 + 6.00 = -2.00D$

$\ell' = 100/-2.00 = -50cm$

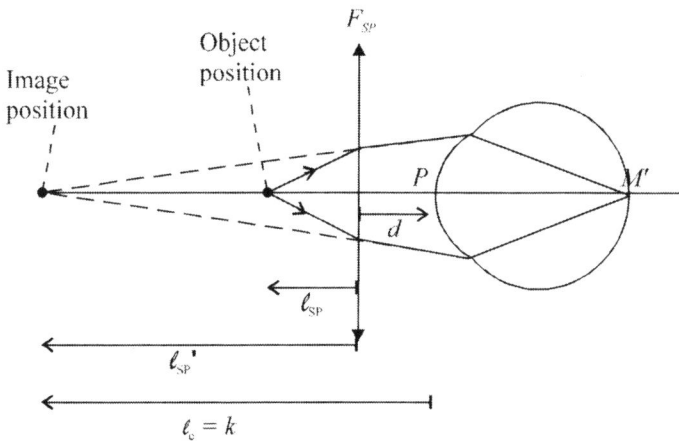

$d = 14mm = 1.4cm$

So from diagram

$k = -51.4cm$

$K = 100/k = 100/-51.4$
$= -1.95D$

Axially ametropic
so $Fe = +60.00$

$\overline{K}' = K + F_e$
$= -1.95 + 60$
$= +58.05D$

$k' = n'/\overline{K}' = (1000 \times 4/3)/58.05 = +22.97mm$

Ocular refraction $= -1.95D$, axial length $= +22.97mm$

This part of the question is the reverse of the first part. The ametropia is given, the object position is required. The far point is the image position.

$K = +1.95D$

$k = 100/1.95 = +51.282cm$

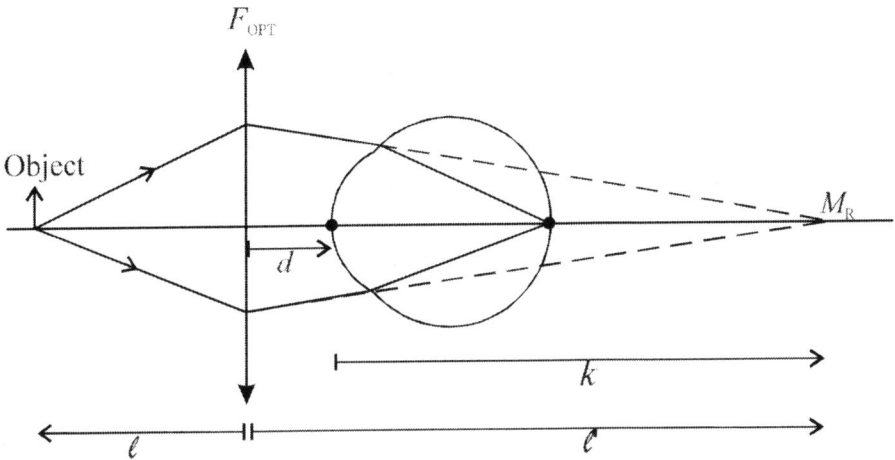

$d = 1.4cm$

So from diagram

$\ell\,' = +52.68cm$

$L' = 100/52.68$
$= +1.90D$

$F = +6.00D$

so $L = 1.90 - 6.00$
$= -4.10D$

The object position $\ell = 100/-4.10$
$= -24.39cm$

60. An emmetropic eye with a reduced surface power of +65.00D views a Snellen chart at 6m. If the letters on this eye's best line produce a retinal image size of –0.0895mm what is the Snellen acuity of this eye?

What is the height of print that this eye could just distinguish at 33.33cm?

Emmetropic eye so $\overline{K}' = F_e = +65.00D$

$h' = -1000(\tan \omega)/\overline{K}'$

So $\tan \omega = -h' \times \overline{K}'/1000$

$h' = -0.0895mm$

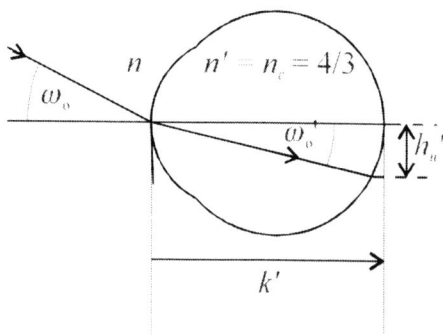

So $\tan \omega_o =$
$-(0.0895) \times 65/1000$
$= 0.0895 \times 0.065$
Object size $h = \ell \times \tan \omega_o$

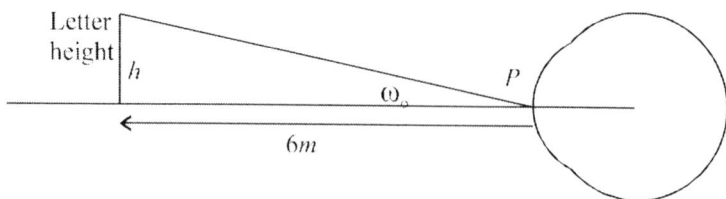

$= 6000 \times 0.0895 \times 0.065$
$= 34.91mm$

So the letters on the Best Line are 34.91mm high.

To find where these letters
subtend 5'

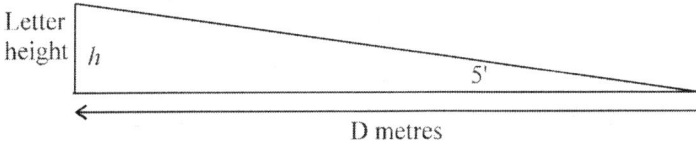

$D = h/\tan 5'$
    $= 34.91/\tan 5 = 24002mm$
    $= 24m$ (approx.)
So the VA is 6/24

The size of print legible at 33.33cm can be calculated either with similar triangles or using $\tan \omega_b$.

By $\tan \omega_b$ and substituting 33.33cm in diagram

$h = 333.3 \times \tan \omega$
  $= 333.3 \times 0.0895 \times 0.065$
  $= 1.94mm$

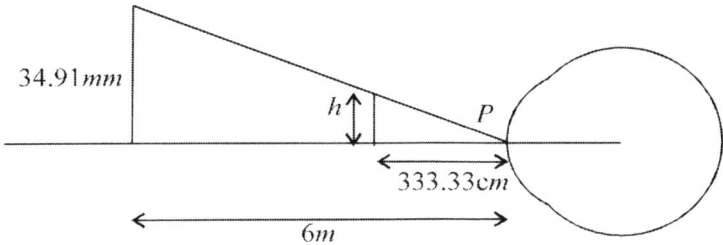

OR
by similar triangles
$h/34.91 = 333.3/6000$
$h = 34.91 \times 333.3/6000$
  $= 1.94mm$

61. An object is situated midway between the eyes and at a distance of 25cm from the line joining the centres of rotation of the two eyes. Calculate the convergence required for a subject with a PD of 68mm to view the object. Give your answer in i) Metre Angles ii) Prism Dioptres iii) Degrees.

The same object is now viewed through +3.00DS lenses placed 20mm in front of the centres of rotation. The lenses are centred for the subject's distance PD. Calculate the convergence required and give your answer in i) Prism Dioptres ii) Degrees.

Object at 25cm, semi-PD is 34mm

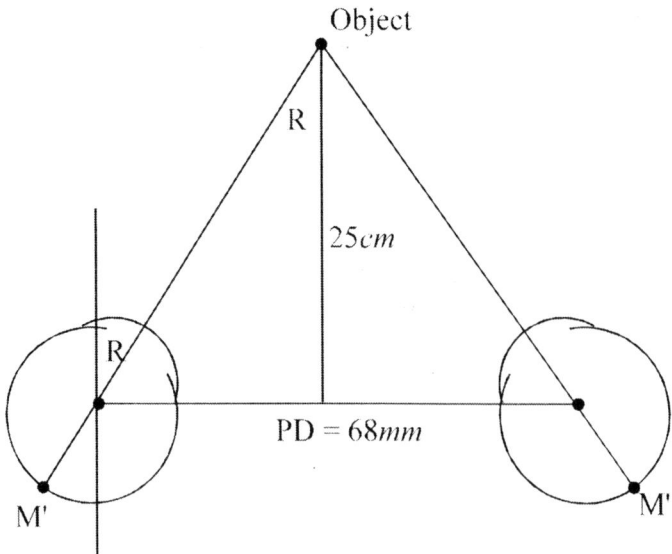

Object

R

25cm

R

PD = 68mm

M'   M'

i) Convergence required is
   $100/25 = 4MA$

ii) To find the angle in prism dioptres
tan R = 34/250 = 0.136
R = 13.6Δ

iii) In degrees
tan R = 0.136 So R = 7° 45'

With the +3.00DS lenses. The image position must be found first.

$\ell = -(25 - 2) = -23cm$ $L = 100/-23 = -4.35D$

$F = +3.00$ So $L' = -4.35 + 3 = -1.35D$

$\ell' = 100/-1.35 = -74.07cm$

From similar triangles in diagram $h'/34 = 740.7/230$
    $h' = 34 \times 740.7/230$
      $= 109.5mm$

i) tan R = $h'/(\ell' + 20)$
  = 109.5/(740.7 + 20)
  = 109.5/760.7
  = 0.144
So R = 14.4Δ

ii) R = 8° 11'

Note that the effect of the lenses is to increase the convergence required.

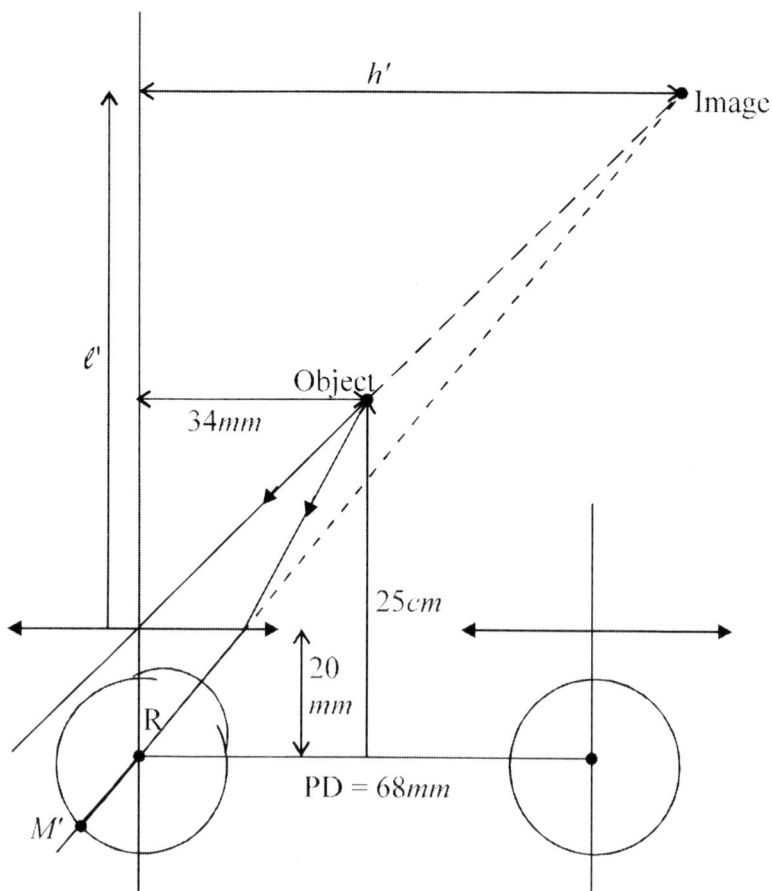

---

62. An eye is corrected for distance vision by $-10.00DS$ lens placed $12mm$ from the reduced surface. If the power of the reduced surface is $+61.50D$ find the axial length of the eye.
The eye views an object $33.33cm$ in front of the spectacle lens. Calculate the spectacle and ocular accommodation used.
If the eye has an amplitude of accommodation of $6.00D$, find the position of the apparent near point.

$F_{SP} = -10.00D$
$d = 12mm = 1.2cm$
To find k' use $\overline{K}' = K + F_e$, so K must be found first.

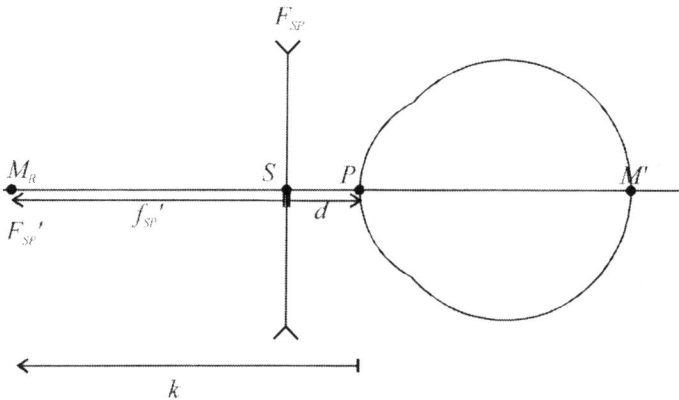

$f'_{SP} = 100/{-10} = -10cm$
From diagram $k = -11.2cm$
$K = 100/{-11.2} = -8.93D$

$F_e = +61.50D$
So $\overline{K}' = -8.93 + 61.50$
$\quad = +52.57D$

$$k' = n'/\overline{K}'$$
$$= (4/3 \times 1000)/52.57$$
$$= +25.36mm$$

Axial length is $+25.36mm$

Object at $33.33cm$, that is $\ell_{SP} = -33.33cm$ So $L_{SP} = -3.00D$

Spectacle accommodation A_{SP} is given by $-L_{SP}$ So $A_{SP} = +3.00D$

As the eye is myopic it is expected that the ocular accommodation will be less than the spectacle accommodation. To find ocular accommodation use $A = K - L_e$

ℓ_e is the distance from the eye of the image formed by the lens.

$L_{SP} = -3.00$ and $F_{SP} = -10.00$ So $L_{SP}' = -3.00 + (-10.00)$
$= -13.00D$
$\ell_{SP}' = 100/L_{SP}' = 100/-13 = -7.69cm$

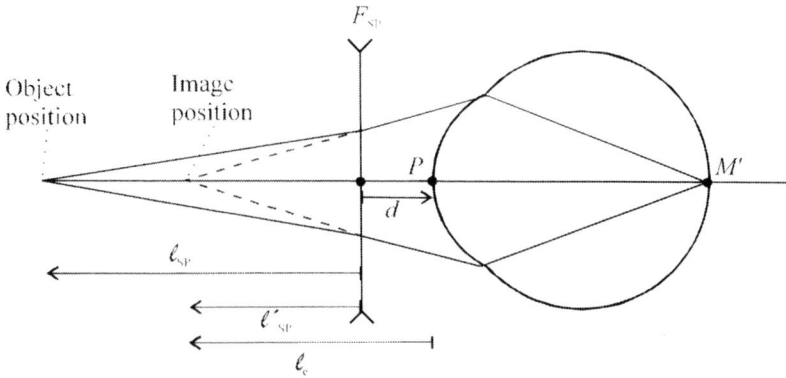

From diagram

$\ell_e = -(7.69 + 1.2)$

$= -8.89cm$

$L_e = 100/-8.89$

$= -11.25D$

$A = -8.93 - (-11.25)$

$= +2.32D$

Ocular accommodation required is $+2.32D$

Amplitude of accommodation is $6.00D$. Finding the position of the apparent near point is the reverse of previous part, that is, A is known and ℓ_{SP} must be found.

Expected value is approx. $100/6 \approx -17cm$. As the lens is negative the actual distance will be closer than this.

$A = 6.00\ D$ and $K = -8.93D$

So re-arranging $A = K - L_e$ gives $L_e = -8.93 - 6.00 = -14.93D$

$\ell_e = 100/-14.93 = -6.70cm$

$d = 1.2cm$ so from diagram $\ell_{SP}' = -5.50cm$

$L_{SP}' = 100/-5.5 = -18.18D$

$L_{SP} = L_{SP}' - F_{SP} = -18.18 - (-10.00) = -8.18D$

So $\ell_{SP} = 100/-8.18 = -12.22cm$

So the apparent near point is $-12.22cm$ from the lens.

63. An eye with refractive ametropia of $+6.50D$ is corrected for distance vision by a lens at $15mm$. It views a $24m$ Snellen letter at a distance of $6m$.

Calculate the size of the Snellen letter object, the axial length of the eye, the power of the spectacle lens, the spectacle magnification and the retinal image size in the corrected eye.

$K = +6.50D$ $d = 15mm = 1.5cm$
Refractive ametropia so $k' = +22.22mm$

A $24m$ Snellen letter subtends 5' at $24m$

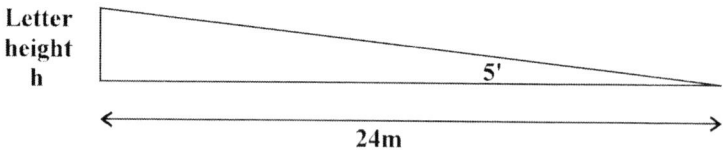

Using diagram

$h = 24,000 \times \tan5'$
$\quad = 34.91mm$

Refractive ametropia so by definition the axial length
$k' = +22.22mm$

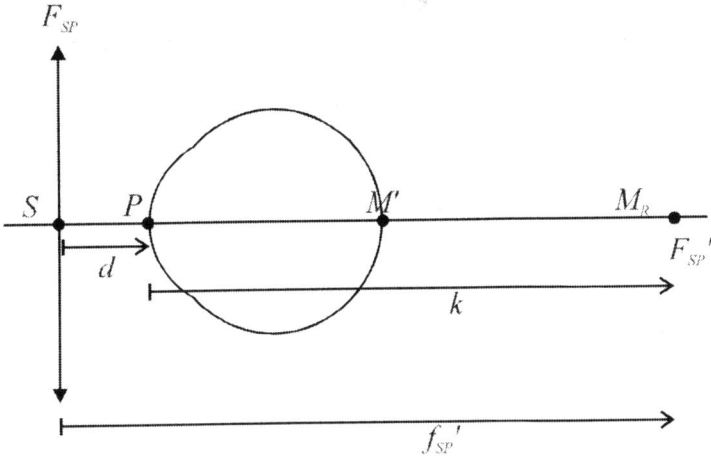

$K = +6.50D$
So $k = 100/6.5$ $d = 1.5cm$
$= +15.38cm$

From diagram
$f_{SP}' = +16.88cm$
$F_{SP} = 100/16.88$
$= +5.92D$

Spectacle magnification
$= K/F_{SP}$
$SM = 6.5/5.92 = 1.098$

The corrected retinal image size h_C' equals $h_u' \times SM$
$h_u' = -(1000 \times \tan \omega)/ \overline{K}'$
$\tan \omega_0 = 34.91/6000$ and $\overline{K}' = +60.00D$
So $h_u' = -(1000 \times 34.91/6000)/60 = -0.097mm$
$h_C' = -0.097 \times 1.098 = -0.107mm$

64. A simple optometer uses a fan chart as the target and a lens of power +3.00DS. Find the positions of the target when measuring the spectacle refraction $-3.00/-2.00 \times 90$ assuming that the spectacle lens would be in the same plane as the optometer lens. What is the direction of the line that appears clear for each target position ?

$$F_{SP} = -3.00/-2.00 \times 90 = -3.00 \times 180/-5.00 \times 90$$

As with all astigmatism problems each meridian must be considered separately.

The image formed by the optometer lens must be at the far point and, as the optometer lens is in the same plane as the spectacle lens this will be at its second principal focus, giving $\ell' = f'_{SP}$.

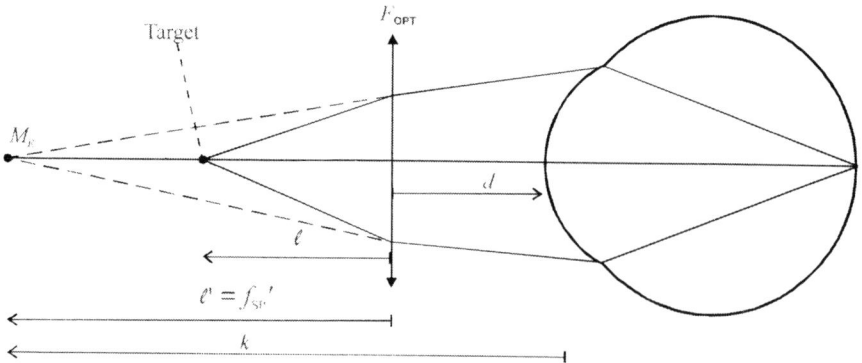

Axis 90

$F_{SP} = -5.00D = L'$
$F_{OPT} = +3.00D$
$L = L' - F_{OPT} = -5 - 3$
$\qquad = -8.00D$

$\ell' = 100/L' = 100/-8$
$= -12.5cm$

The target position for axis 90 will be $-12.5cm$ from the optometer lens.

The clear line on the fan chart will be parallel to the axis, that is the vertical line.

Axis 180

$F_{SP} = -3.00D = L'$
$F_{OPT} = +3.00D$

$L' = -3 - 3 = -6.00D$

$\ell' = 100/-6 = -16.67cm$

The target position for axis 180 will be $-16.67cm$ from the optometer lens.

The clear line will be horizontal

65. An eye is corrected for distance vision by a lens at 11.7*mm* from the reduced surface. If the power of the eye is +62.50*D* and the axial length is +22.99*mm*, find the power of the spectacle lens.

A 1*cm* high object is placed 45*cm* from the lens. Calculate the ocular accommodation required and the retinal image size.

$k' = +22.99mm$ $\overline{K}' = n'/k' = (1000 \times 4/3)/22.99 = +58.00D$

$F_e = +62.50D$ So $K = \overline{K}' - F_e = 58.00 - 62.50 = -4.50D$

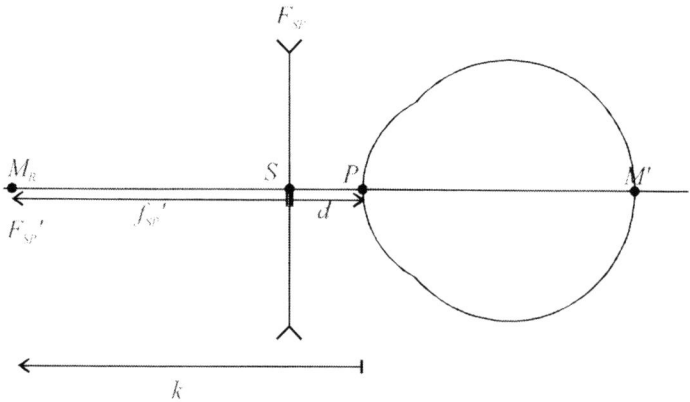

$K = -4.50D$

$k = 100/-4.50$
$= -22.22cm$
$d = 11.7mm = 1.17cm$

From diagram

$f_{SP}' = -21.05cm$

$F_{SP}' = 1/f_{SP}' = 100/-21.05$
$\qquad = -4.75D$

So the power of the spectacle lens is $-4.75D$

The object is at $-35cm$ and the eye is myopic, so the expected amount of accommodation required will be a little less than $3.00D$.

To find the ocular accommodation required use $A = K - L_e$

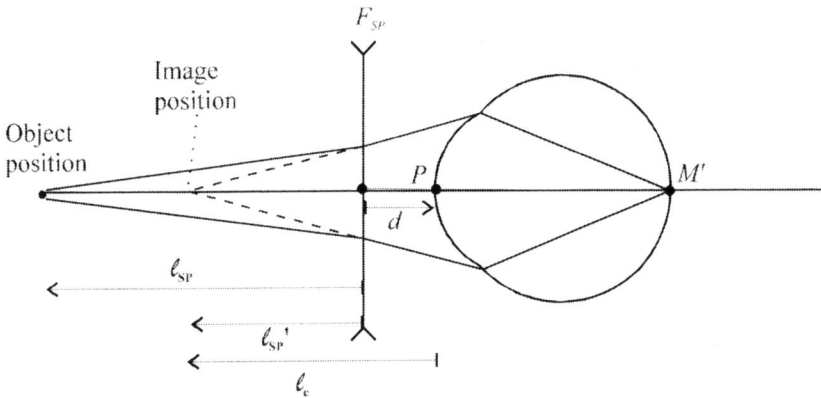

$\ell_{SP} = -35cm$
So $L_{SP} = 100/-35 = -2.86D$

$F_{SP}' = -4.75D$
$L_{SP}' = L_{SP} + F_{SP}'$
$\qquad = -2.86 + (-4.75)$

$$= -7.61D$$
$$\ell_{SP}' = 100/-7.61$$
$$= -13.14cm$$

From diagram

$$\ell_e = -14.31cm$$
$$L_e = 100/-14.31 \quad d = 1.17cm$$
$$= -6.99D$$

$$A = -4.50 - (-6.99)$$
$$= +2.49D$$

To find the retinal image size use the magnification of the lens and the magnification of the eye.

$$h'' = h \times m_{SP} \times m_e = h \times L_{SP}/L_{SP}' \times L_e/\overline{K}'$$

$$= 10 \times -2.86/-7.61 \times -6.99/58.00 = -0.453mm$$

So the accommodation required is $2.49D$ and the retinal image size is $-0.453mm$

66. A spot of light at *6m* is observed binocularly with 5Δ base up in front of the right eye. What is the apparent separation of the two images ? Which eye sees the higher image ?

If the subject has 8Δ exophoria what will be the horizontal separation of the two images? Draw a diagram with dimensions to show the relative positions of the two images.

The strong vertical prism cannot be overcome by the fusional reserves so the subject will experience diplopia.

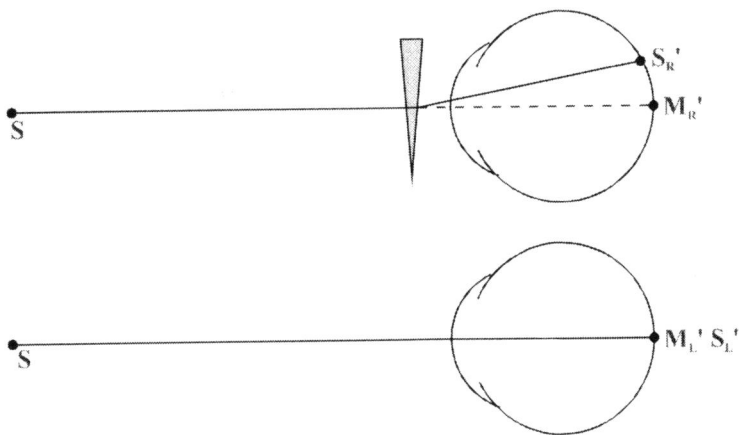

The two eyes (seen from the side) looking at the spotlight S with a strong base up prism in front of the right eye. The image in the right eye is shifted upwards across the retina.

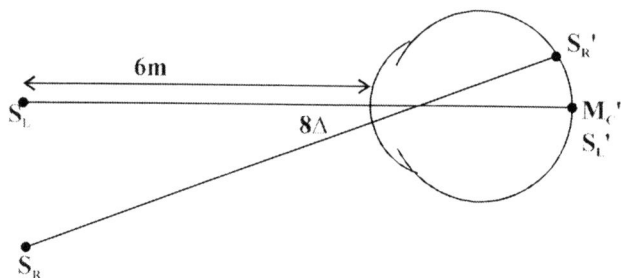

The cyclopean eye (side view) showing the relative positions of the two images.

From the diagrams it can be seen that the image seen by the right eye is below that seen by the left eye.

The apparent separation of the two images can be calculated using the deviation produced by the prism.

Separation = 5 × 6 = 30*cm*.

As the subject has diplopia the eyes are dissociated and will take up their heterophoric position, that is diverged by 8Δ. From the following diagrams the horizontal positions of the two images can be seen.

The two eyes seen from above.

For convenience the exophoria has been shown in the right eye, although it could also have been shown in the left eye, or split between the two eyes.

The cyclopean eye, showing that image seen by the right eye is on the left of that seen by the left eye.

Separation = $8 \times 6 = 48cm$

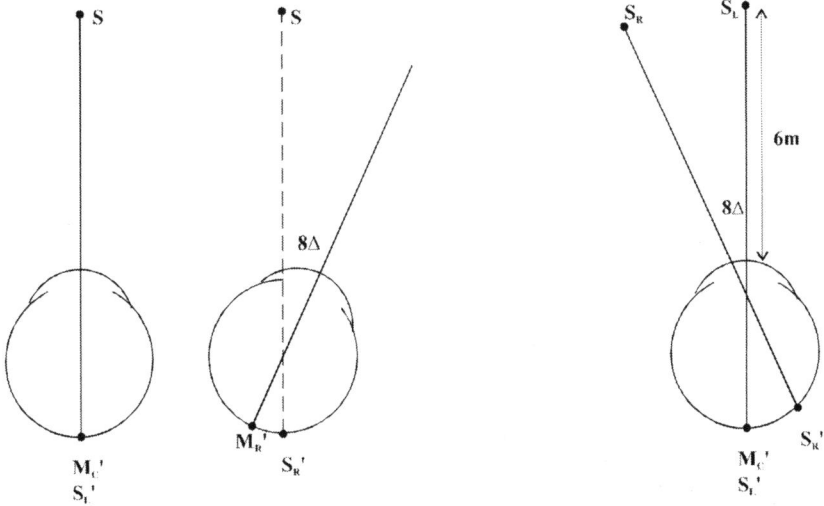

This shows the appearance of the two images as seen by the subject.

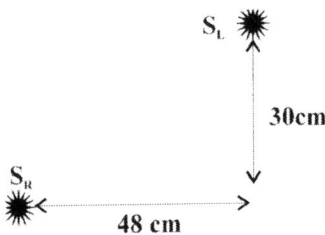

67. A subject can just read a 52*mm* high Snellen letter at 6*m*. Calculate the Minimum Angle of Resolution (in minutes), the decimal acuity and the Snellen acuity.

$h = 52mm \quad \ell = 6m$

The thickness of each limb of the letter will be 52/5 = 10.4*mm*

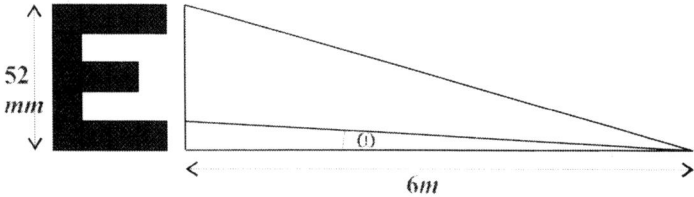

So the Minimum Angle of Resolution (ω) is found from
Tan ω = 10.4/6000
$$\omega = 6'$$
Acuity is $1/\omega = 1/6 = 0.1667$ This is the decimal acuity

Snellen acuity is given by $6/6 \times 1/6 = 6/36$

Or using from the diagram below
The letter subtends 5' at 52/tan5' = 35753*mm* $\approx$ 36*m*

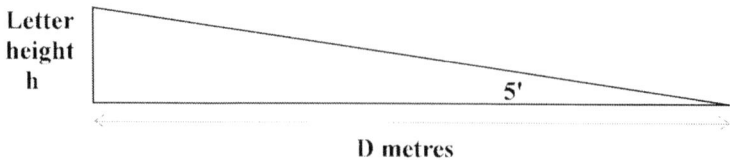

So the VA is 6/36

68. [a] A subject with a PD of 66*mm* can just detect the separation of two objects which are at distances of 105*m* and 110*m*. Calculate the stereoacuity in seconds.
[b]Explain what is meant by the limit to stereopsis. Calculate this limit for the subject in [a].

PD = 66*mm* ℓ = 105m and dℓ = 5m

SA is given by (PD × dℓ)/ℓ^2. Remember that all distances must be in the same units.

$$SA = \frac{66 \times 5000}{105000^2} = 2.993 \times 10^{-5} \, radians$$
$$= 6.17 \, seconds$$

When an object is so far away that its binocular parallax is less that the subject's stereoacuity, its separation from another further object cannot be detected, no matter how great the separation.
For the subject in [a] the stereoacuity is 6.17" so to have a binocular parallax of 6.17" an object must be at a distance of -

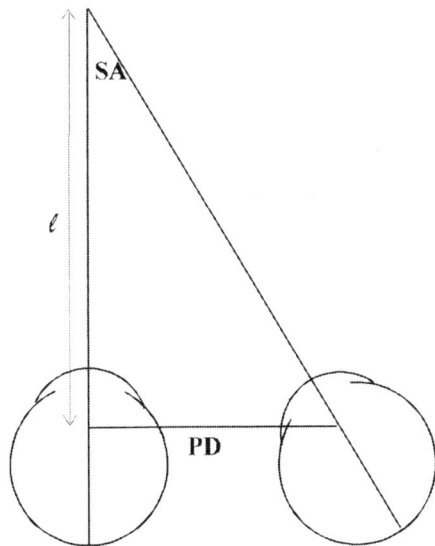

$$\ell = PD/\tan 6.17''$$

$$= \frac{66}{2.991 \times 10^{-5}} = 2206619.9mm = 2207m$$

So the relative position of objects further than this distance [approx. 2*km*] cannot be detected by stereopsis. However, many of the monocular clues such as overlapping and aerial perspective will still operate.

69. Two subjects each have a stereoacuity of 12" One has a PD of 66*m* and the other has a PD of 60*mm*. They view two small objects, one of which is 15*m* away and the other a little further. Find the minimum separation of the objects for each subject to be able to detect which object is the further away.

The relationship $SA = PD.d\ell/\ell^2$ needs to be rearranged to determine $d\ell$.

This gives $d\ell = SA \times \ell^2/PD$

Subject 1 SA = 12", PD = 66*mm*, ℓ = 15*m*

$d\ell = \tan 12" \times 15\,000^2/66 = 198mm$

Subject 2 SA = 12", PD = 60*mm*, ℓ = 15*m*

$d\ell = \tan 12" \times 15\,000^2/60 = 218mm$

So the separation of the two objects needs to be 198*mm* for the subject with a PD of 66*mm* and 218*mm* for the subject with the PD of 60*mm*. This demonstrates that with a larger PD smaller separations can be detected.

70. A reduced eye has an axial length of $+19.80mm$ and a power of $+57.34D$. What is its ocular refraction ?

If the pupil diameter is $5mm$, calculate the blur circle size formed by a distant point object.

What would be the retinal image size of a distant object subtending 5Δ?

What lens placed at $12mm$ from the reduced surface would correct this eye for distance vision ?

Calculate the retinal image size formed in the corrected eye by the same distant object.

$k' = +19.80mm$ So

$F_e = +57.34D$ Using $K' = K' - F_e$ gives
$K = 67.34 - 57.34 = +10.00D$
$\therefore$ The ocular refraction is $+10.00D$

$p = 5mm$
As the object is distant

$y = p\left|\dfrac{K}{K'}\right|$

$y = 5\left[\dfrac{10.00}{67.34}\right]$

$y = 0.7425mm$

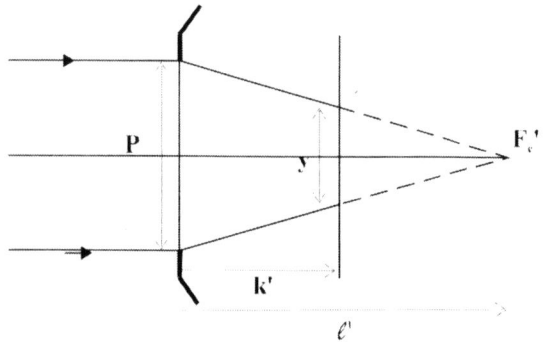

The blur circle size is $0.7425mm$

$w = 5\Delta$ so tan w = 5/100 = 0.05

$$h'_u = -\frac{1000 \times \tan w_0}{\overline{K}'} = -\frac{1000 \times 0.05}{67.34} = -0.7425mm$$

The total retinal image size is given by $h'_u + y = 0.7425 + 0.7425$ = 1.485mm.

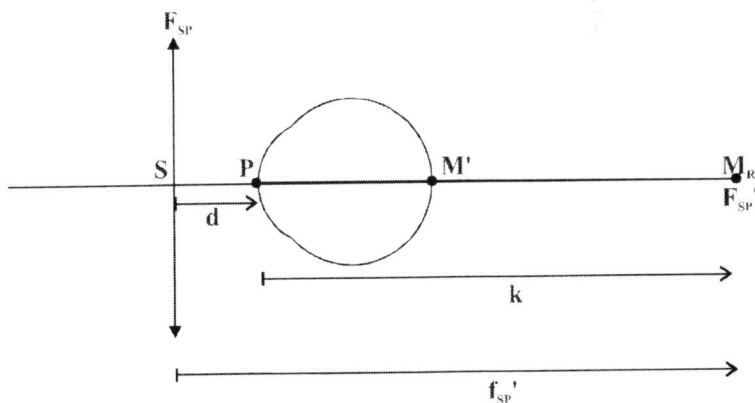

$K = +10.00D$ So k = 100/10.00 = +10.00cm d = 12mm = 1.2cm

From diagram

$f_{SP}' = +11.2cm$

$F_{SP} = 100/11.2$
      $= +8.93D$

The distance correcting lens is +8.93D

Corrected retinal image size is given by $h'_u \times SM$
SM = K/F_{SP} = 10.00/8.93 = 1.12

$h'_C = -0.7425 \times 1.12 = -0.832mm$

The corrected retinal image size is $-0.832mm$

> **71.** An eye with an amplitude of accommodation of 3.00D is corrected for distance by +6.00DS placed 12mm from the reduced surface. Calculate the positions of the apparent far and near points.
> This eye is now given a reading addition of +3.50D. Find the new positions of the apparent far and near points and the range of clear vision obtained

The apparent far point is the object position which will form a clear retinal image in an unaccommodated eye with a lens. As the lens that is worn here is the distance correcting lens the apparent far point is at ∞

To find the apparent near point it is necessary to know the position of the real near point, this is found using $Amp = K - B$.

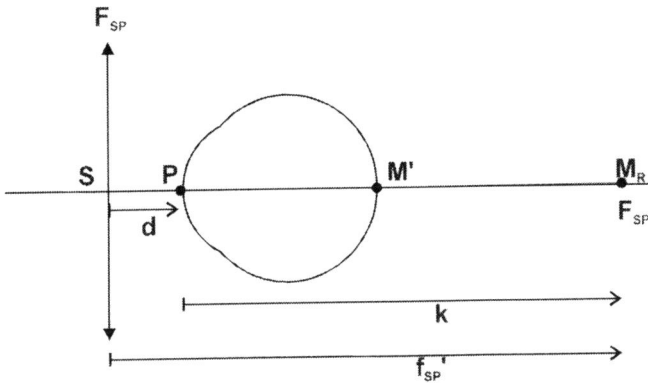

To find K

$F_{SP} = +6.00D$
So $f_{SP}' = 100/6 = +16.67cm$

135

$d = 12$mm $= 1.2cm$

From diagram $k = +15.47cm$

$K = 100/15.47 = +6.46D$

$Amp = 3.00D$

So $B = K - Amp$

$= 6.46 - 3.00 = +3.46D$

$b = 100/3.46 = +28.90cm$

The image formed by the lens is at the real near point, that is at $+28.90cm$ from the eye, which is $+30.10cm$ from the lens (see diagram below).

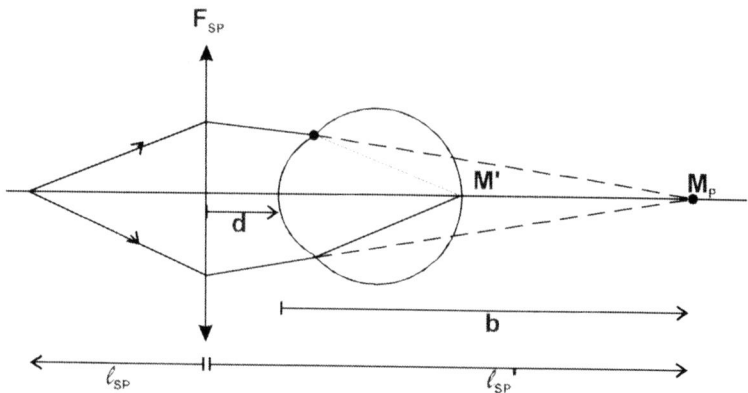

$\ell_{SP}' = +30.10cm$

$L_{SP}' = 100/30.10$

$= +3.32D$

$F_{SP} = +6.00D$

So $L_{SP} = 3.32 - 6$
$= -2.68D$

$\ell_{SP} = 100/-2.68$
$= -37.31cm$

The apparent near point is $-37.31cm$ from the lens.

Reading addition of $+3.50D$, so the lens power is now $+9.50D$

$k = +15.47cm$ and $\ell_{SP}' = +16.67cm$

$L_{SP}' = +6.00$ So $L_{SP} = 6.00 - 9.50 = -3.50D$

$\ell_{SP} = 100/-3.5 = -28.57cm$

This is the apparent far point with the reading lens

$b = +28.90cm$ and $\ell_{SP}' = +30.10cm$

$L_{SP}' = +3.32D$ So $L_{SP} = 3.32 - 9.50 = -6.18D$

Apparent near point is $100/-6.18 = -16.18cm$

The range of clear vision with the reading prescription is from
-28.57cm to $-16.18cm = 12.39cm$

72. [a] Define spectacle magnification.

[b] The power of the reduced surface of a refractively ametropic eye is +52D in the horizontal meridian and +55D in the vertical meridian. Determine the prescription of the thin correcting lens at 12mm.

[c] Calculate the spectacle magnification.

[d] The above eye views a distant spherical object of angular diameter 3°. Calculate the size of the retinal image in the uncorrected and corrected eye. Sketch the form of the retinal image in the latter case.

[e] The uncorrected eye in [b] views a distant thin wire square with vertical and horizontal sides, the plane of the square being perpendicular to the visual axis. Sketch the form of the retinal image if the eye applies

(i) 5.00D,

(ii) 6.50D and

(iii) 8.00D of ocular accommodation.

[a] Spectacle magnification is defined as the ratio of the corrected retinal image size to the basic size of the retinal image of the same object in the uncorrected eye. That is $SM = h_c'/h_U'$

[b] Refractively ametropic so k' is standard thus $\overline{K}' = +60.00D$

Axis 90

$F_c = +52.00D$

$K = \overline{K}' - F_c$

$\quad = 60 - 52$

$\quad = +8.00D$

$k = 100/8$

$\quad = +12.50cm$

Axis 180

$F_c = +55.00D$

$\quad\quad K = 60 - 55$

$\quad = +5.00D$

$k = 100/5$

$\quad = +20cm$

138

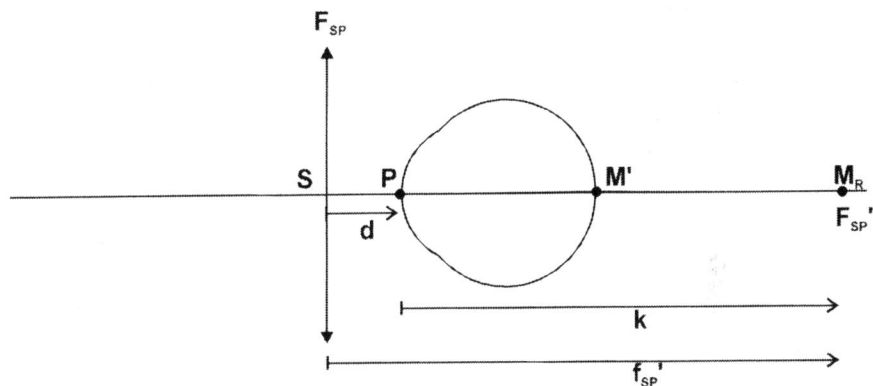

$d = 12mm = 1.2cm$ $d = 1.2cm$

From diagram

$f_{SP}' = +13.70cm$ $f_{SP}' = +21.20cm$

$F_{SP} = +7.30D$ $F_{SP} = +4.72D$

So the lens power is $+7.30 \times 90/+4.72 \times 180$

$$= +7.30/-2.58 \times 180$$

[c] $SM = K/F_{SP}$

   $= 8/7.30$ $SM = 5/4.72$

   $= 1.096$ $= 1.059$

[d] $h_U' = -(1000 \times \tan w)/\overline{K}'$. This is the same for both meridians as K' and w_o are the same.

$h_U' = -(1000 \times \tan 3°)/60 = -0.873mm$

$h_C' = h_U' \times SM$

$$= -0.873 \times 1.096 \qquad h_c' = -0.873 \times 1.059$$
$$= -0.957mm \qquad\qquad = -0.925mm$$

So the corrected retinal image is
0.957mm along the horizontal and
0.925mm vertically,

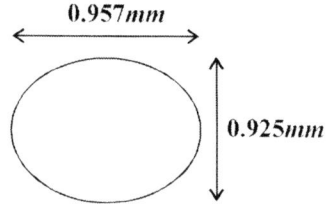

0.957mm

0.925mm

[e] In the uncorrected eye using no accommodation both focal lines
are behind the retina

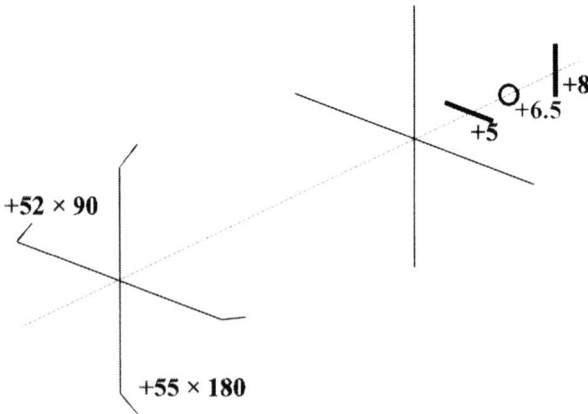

+8

O +6.5

+5

+52 × 90

+55 × 180

(i) When 5.00*D* of accommodation is used, the front focal line is brought onto the retina. The retinal image is a square made up of horizontal lines

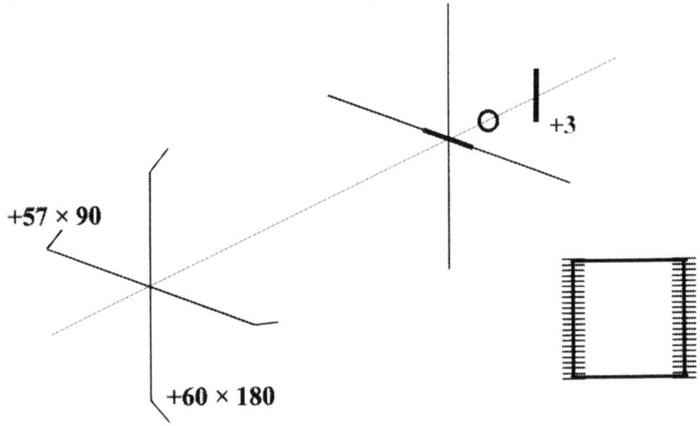

+57 × 90

+60 × 180

+3

(ii) 6.50*D* of accommodation brings the circle of least confusion onto the retina so the retinal image is made up of circular blurs.

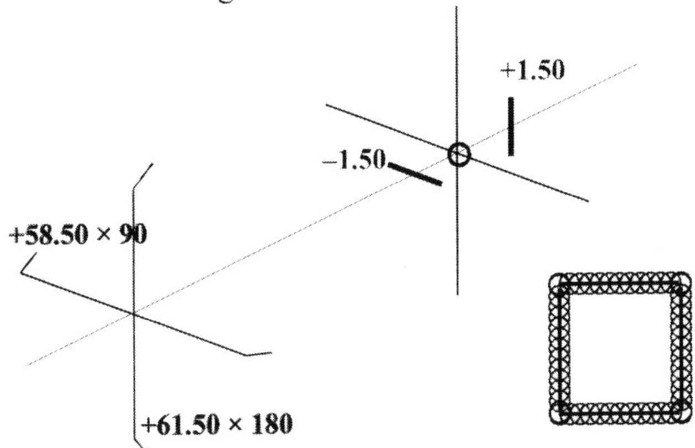

+58.50 × 90

+61.50 × 180

+1.50

−1.50

(iii) 8.00D puts
the second
(vertical) focal
line on the retina.

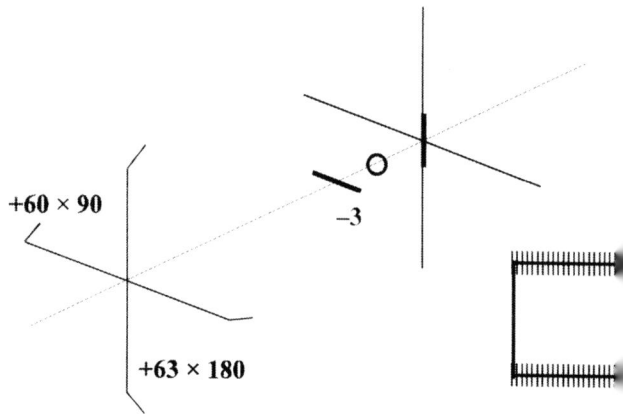

+60 × 90

+63 × 180

−3

73. An axially ametropic eye is corrected for distance vision by – 8.00D placed 14*mm* from the reduced surface P. This eye is rendered aphakic and has a corneal radius of 7.8*mm*. Assuming the cornea to be situated 1.68*mm* in front of P, find the power of the new spectacle lens required in the same plane as the original lens.

Find the spectacle magnifications required for the phakic and aphakic eyes assuming the correcting lenses are thin. Calculate the size of the retinal images in both cases for a distant object subtending 2°.

If the aphakic correcting lens is considered to be thick, calculate the spectacle magnification that it will produce. Assume $t = 9mm$, $n = 1.523$ and $F_1 = +10.00D$.

In order to find out the ametropia of the aphakic eye its axial length is required, so the first step is to find the axial length of the phakic eye.

Diag. [i]

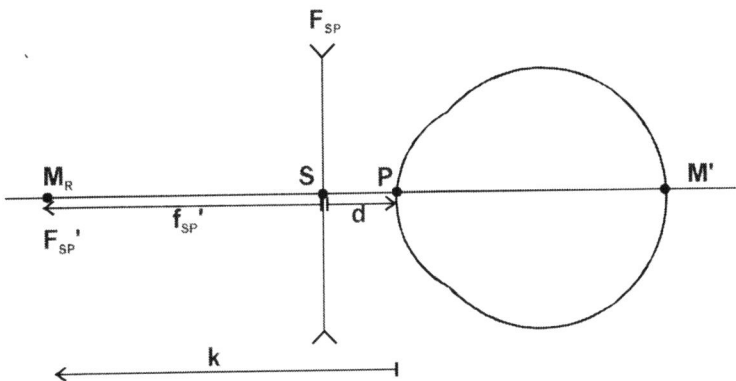

$F_{SP} = -8.00D$
$f_{SP}' = 100/-8$
$= -12.50cm$

$d = 14mm = 1.4cm$

From diagram [i]

$k = -13.90cm$
$K = 100/-13.90cm$
$= -7.19D$

Axial ametropia so $F_e = +60.00D$

$\overline{K}' = -7.19 + 60 = +52.81D$

$k' = 4/3 \times 1000/52.81$
$= +25.25mm$

In aphakic eye (see diagram [ii])

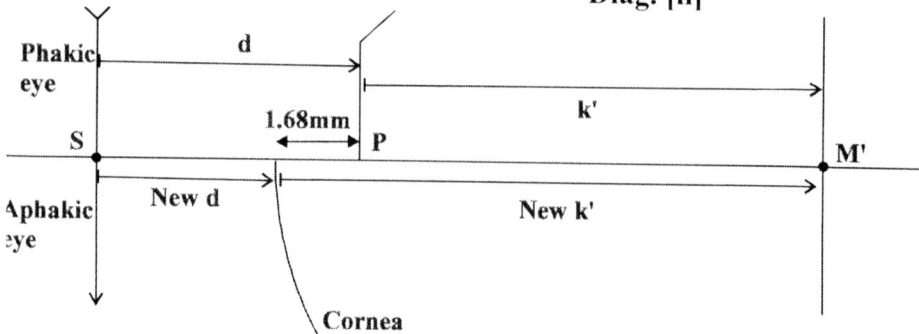

Diag. [ii]

$k' = 25.25 + 1.68 = +26.93mm$
$\overline{K}' = 4/3 \times 1000/26.93 = +49.51D$
$r = +7.8mm$

So $F_e = \dfrac{1000 \times (\frac{4}{3} - 1)}{7.8} = +42.74D$

$K = 49.51 - 42.74 = +6.77D$

To find F_{SP} in aphakic eye

$k = 100/6.77 = +14.77cm$

Diag. [iii]

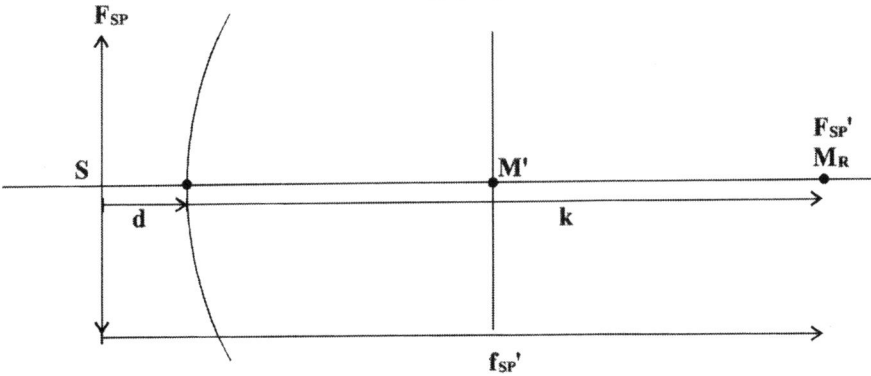

From diagram [ii]

New $d = 14 - 1.68$

$= 12.32mm \qquad = 1.232cm$

From diagram [iii] $f_{SP}' = 14.77 + 1.232$
$= +16.00cm$

$F_{SP} = 100/16 = +6.25D$

Phakic eye $SM = K/F_{SP}$
$= -7.19/-8 = 0.899$

Aphakic eye $SM = 6.77/6.25$
$\quad = 1.083$

To find retinal image size use $h_C' = h_U' \times SM$

In phakic eye $h_U' = -1000 \times \tan 2°/ 52.81 = -0.661mm$

$h_C' = -0.661 \times 0.899 = -0.594mm$

In aphakic eye $h_U' = -1000 \times \tan 2°/ 49.51 = -0.705mm$

$h_C' = -0.705 \times 1.083 = -0.764mm$

Note the retinal image size is approximately 30% larger in the aphakic eye than it was in the myopic eye before the crystalline lens was removed.

Thick lens $\quad t = 9mm \quad\quad n = 1.523 \quad\quad F_1 = +10.00D$

$$SM = \frac{1}{\left(1 - [^t/_n]F_1\right)} \times \frac{1}{\left(1 - dF_v'\right)}$$

$$= \frac{1}{\left(1 - [0.009/1.523]10\right)} \times \frac{1}{\left(1 - 0.01232 \times 6.25\right)}$$

$$= 1.063 \times 1.083$$

$$= 1.151$$

---

74. [a] A myopic reduced eye can be corrected by a $-6.00D$ thin lens at $13mm$. If the axial length is $24.40mm$ and $n' = 4/3$ calculate the power of the reduced surface.
[b] If the ocular amplitude of accommodation is $2.25D$ and two-thirds of this is to be used for comfortable near vision, find the Add required to read at $40cm$ from the spectacle plane (which is $13mm$ from the eye). Express your answer to the nearest $0.25D$.
[c] Relative to the thin lens obtained in [b] where are the artificial far and near points ?

---

[a] $F_{SP} = -6.00D$ $f_{SP}' = 100/-6 = -16.67cm$

$d = 13mm = 1.3cm$

Diagram [i]

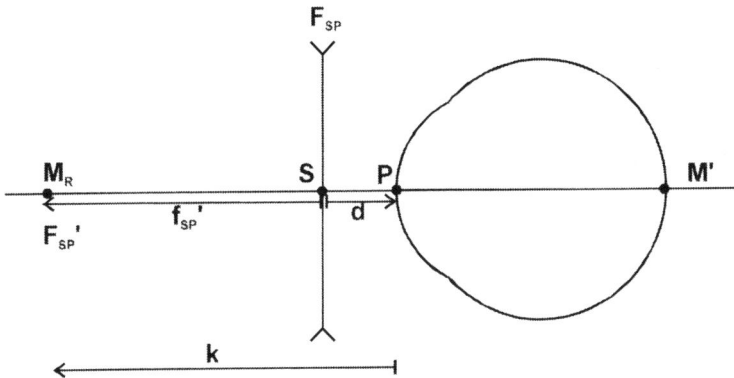

Using diagram [i]

$k = -17.97cm$

$K = 100/-17.97$
$\quad = -5.56D$

$k' = 24.4mm$

So $\overline{K}' = \dfrac{1000 \times \frac{4}{3}}{24.4} = 54.64D$

$F_e = \overline{K}' - K$

$= 54.64 - (-5.56) = +60.20D$

The power of the reduced surface is $+60.20D$

[b] This problem is unusual because it is the lens power that is unknown. The object position is given and the image position can be found, so from this the lens power is calculated.

$\ell_{SP} = -40cm \quad L_{SP} = -2.50D$

To find ℓ_{SP}' it is necessary to calculate ℓ_e using $A = K - L_e$

$Amp = 2.25D$ If 2/3 of this is to be used $A = +1.50D$
$\quad L_e = K - A = -5.56 - 1.50 = -7.06D$

Diagram [ii]

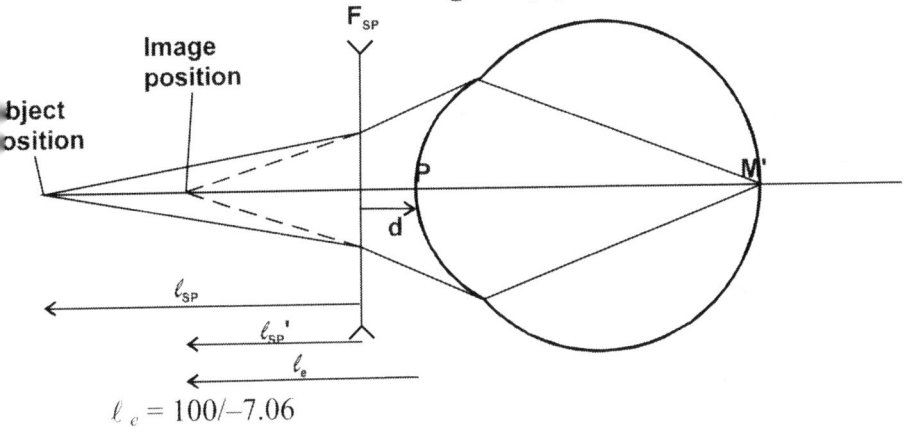

$$\ell_e = 100/-7.06$$
$$= -14.16cm$$

From Diag. [ii]

$$\ell_{SP}' = -12.86cm$$

$$L_{SP}' = 100/-12.86$$
$$= -7.78D$$

So
$$F_{SP} = L_{SP}' - L_{SP}$$
$$= -7.78 - (-2.50)$$
$$= -5.28D$$

The lens required for near vision at $40cm$ is $-5.28D$

As the distance lens is $-6.00D$ the Add is $+0.72D = +0.75D$ (to nearest $0.25D$)

[c] To find the artificial far point, the accommodation is fully relaxed so the image formed by the lens is at the far point.

$\ell_{SP}' = -16.67cm \quad L_{SP}' = -6.00D$

$F_{SP} = -5.28 \quad So \ L_{SP} = -0.72D$

$\ell_{SP} = 100/-0.72 = -138.89cm \quad$ This is the artificial far point

To find the artificial near point all the accommodation is being used.
$L_e = K - A = -5.56 - 2.25 = -7.81D$

$\ell_e = 100/-7.81 = -12.80cm$ so using Diag.[ii]

$\ell_{SP}' = -11.50cm$

$L_{SP}' = 100/-11.50 = -8.70D$

$L_{SP} = -8.70 - (-5.28) = -3.42D$

$\ell_{SP} = 100/-3.42 = -29.24cm \quad$ This is the artificial near point

---

75. [a] A thin +12.00*D* lens is placed 8*cm* in front of an unaccommodated reduced eye. The retinal image is clear when an object is placed 5*cm* in front of the lens. Find the vergence at the eye and explain why this is equal to the eye's ocular refraction. (Use 3 decimal places for all intermediate steps and the final answer.)

[b] Calculate the power of the thin correcting lens at 10*mm* and find the ocular accommodation required when the corrected eye has a clear retinal image of an object at one-third of a metre from the lens.

[c] If the eye in [b] accommodates a further 1.5D, where is the object for a clear retinal image?

---

[a] A clear retinal image is being produced but the object is not at infinity, so the lens is not the distance correcting lens. The object is only 5*cm* from the lens and the lens-eye distance is 8*cm*, so this problem can be treated as an optometer question.

$$\ell = -5cm \quad L = 100/(-5) = -20.00D$$

$$F_{OPT} = +12.00D \quad L' = -20.00 + 12.00 = -8.00D$$

$$\ell' = 100/-8.00 = -12.50cm$$

Diag. [i]

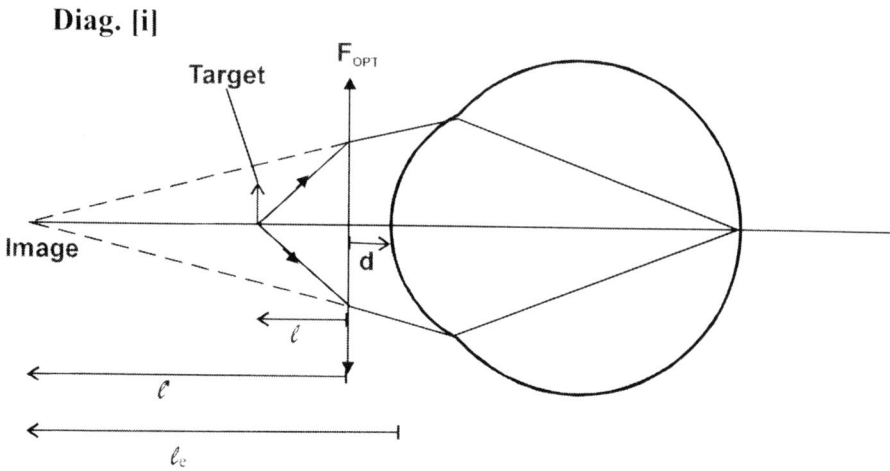

$d = 8cm$ so using Diag. [i]

$\ell_e = -20.50cm$ $L_e = 100/-20.50 = -4.88D$

The vergence reaching the eye is $-4.88D$. As the eye is unaccommodated the image formed by the lens must be at the eye's far point in order to produce a clear retinal image,

Vergence at eye = ocular refraction

so $\ell_e = k$ and $L_e = K$.

[b] $k = -20.50cm$ $d = 10mm = 1cm$

Diag. [ii]

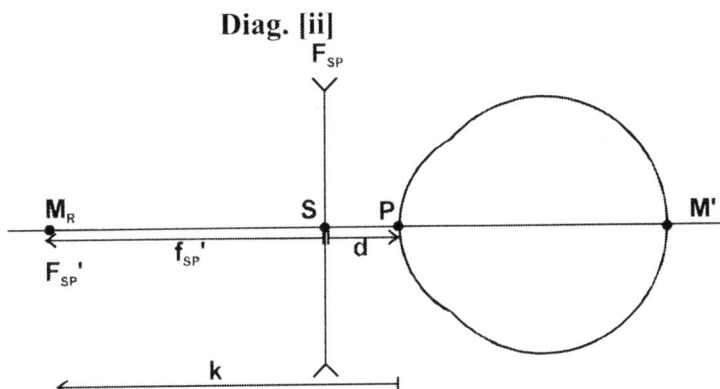

Using Diag. [ii]

$f_{SP}' = -19.5cm$

$F_{SP} = 100/-19.5$
         $= -5.13D$

The distance correcting lens is $-5.13D$

$\ell_{SP} = -1/3m$
$L_{SP} = -3.00D$

$F_{SP} = -5.13D$

$L_{SP}' = -5.13 - 3 = -8.13D$

To find ocular accommodation use $A = K - L_e$

Diag. [iii]

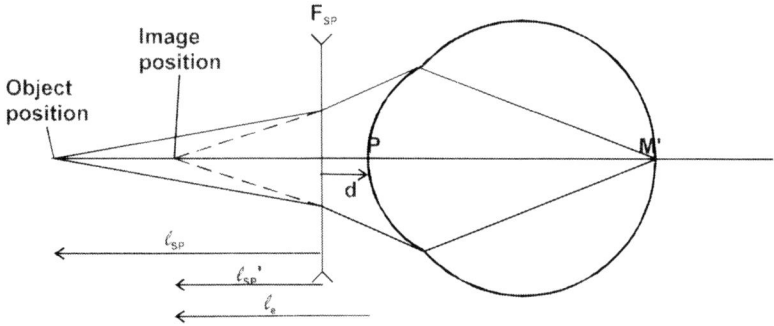

$\ell_{SP}' = 100/-8.13 = -12.30cm$

$d = 1cm$

so using Diag. [iii]

$\ell_e = -13.30cm$

$L_e = 100/-13.30$
$\quad = -7.52D$

$A = K - L_e$
$\quad = -4.88 - (-7.52)$
$\quad = +2.64D$

The ocular accommodation required is $+2.64D$

[c] This part of the question is the reverse of part [b], that is, the accommodation is given but the object position is unknown.

If the eye accommodates by a further 1.50D the ocular accommodation will be +4.14D.

$$L_e = K - A = -4.88 - 4.14 = -9.02D$$

$$\ell_e = 100/-9.02 = -11.09cm$$

Using Diag [iii]

$$\ell_{SP}' = -10.09cm$$

$$L_{SP}' = 100/-10.09 = -9.91D$$

$$L_{SP} = -9.91 - (-5.13) = -4.78D$$

$$\ell_{SP} = -20.92cm$$

The object position is $-20.92cm$ from the lens.